the

NATURAL
MENOPAUSE
METHOD

KAREN NEWBY

To my wonderful circle of women
who navigate womanhood with me
— where would I be without you?

Pavilion
An imprint of HarperCollins*Publishers*
1 London Bridge Street
London SE1 9GF

www.harpercollins.co.uk

HarperCollins*Publishers*
Macken House, 39/40 Mayor Street Upper
Dublin 1, D01 C9W8
Ireland

10 9 8 7 6 5 4 3

First published in Great Britain by
Pavilion, an imprint of HarperCollinsPublishers Ltd
2022

ISBN 978-1-911682-23-3

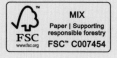

FSC
www.fsc.org

MIX
Paper | Supporting
responsible forestry
FSC™ C007454

This book is produced from independently
certified FSC™ paper to ensure responsible forest
management. For more information visit:
www.harpercollins.co.uk/green

Reproduction by Mission Productions Ltd.

Printed and bound in China by RR Donnelley APS

Commissioning Editor: Cara Armstrong
Editor: Ellen Sandford O'Neill
Copy Editor: Mandy Greenfield
Design Manager: Nicky Collings
Layout Designer: Hannah Naughton
Illustrator: Alja Horvat

Disclaimer: The information in this book is provided
as an information resource only and is not to be used
or relied on for any diagnostic, treatment or medical
purpose. All health issues should be discussed with
your GP and/or other qualified medical professional.

the

NATURAL
MENOPAUSE
METHOD

*a nutritional guide
to perimenopause and
beyond*

KAREN NEWBY

⌐ PAVILION ¬

"

WHEN A WOMAN DECIDES TO CHANGE, EVERYTHING CHANGES AROUND HER.

EUFROSINA CRUZ,
MEXICAN POLITICIAN, FEMALE EQUALITY ACTIVIST
AND INDIGENOUS RIGHTS CAMPAIGNER

"

Contents

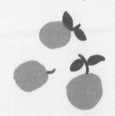

INTRODUCTION

I see time and again in my practice the massive effect that food can have on the symptoms of perimenopause and beyond, which is what I want to share with you in this book. My BSc in Nutritional Medicine was heavy on the biochemistry (I remember thinking, 'When are we going to get to the food bit?'), but it's important to me to present the evidence-based research behind the food and lifestyle interventions that I talk about. I think we benefit from knowing WHY this is all happening. Nutritional therapy in my one-to-one clinic focuses on you as an individual, acknowledging that we all experience menopause differently. So there will be some parts of this book that will resonate more with you than others, and as your symptoms change, you can see this book as a companion, helpful to have close to hand. Therapeutic food has a profound effect on my clients, and I hope that after reading this book and making small but sustainable shifts, you will experience this too.

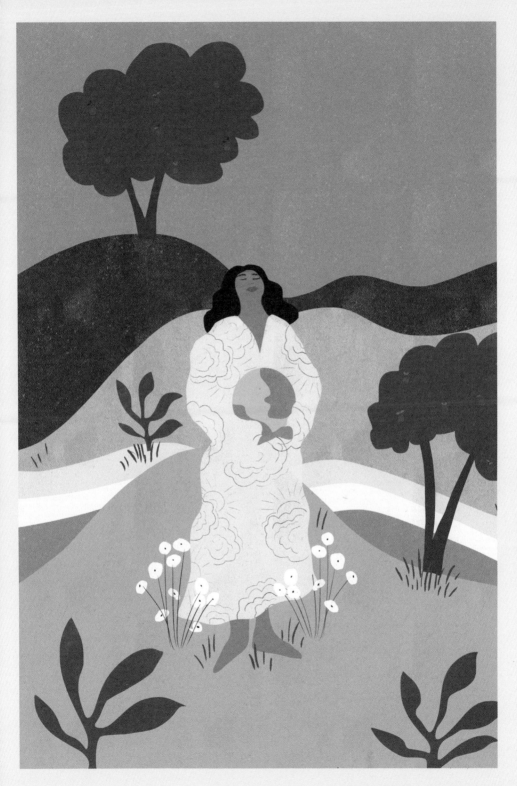

PART ONE

What is going on in my body?

"

WE DELIGHT IN THE BEAUTY OF THE BUTTERFLY BUT RARELY ADMIT THE CHANGES IT HAS GONE THROUGH TO ACHIEVE THAT BEAUTY.

MAYA ANGELOU,
POET AND ACTIVIST

"

how this book will help

As much as we'd all love menopause to be a positive transition, if we're suffering from hot sweats, weight gain, brain fog, extreme fatigue or simply don't like what we see in the mirror, it's not going to be the positive journey that we'd like it to be. But help is at hand in the form of food...and no form of dieting, I promise (I can't bear that side of my industry!) – even if you are suffering from weight around your middle (see page 52). Diets don't work, and they set us (mainly women) up to fail. Food has the power to help us through this entirely natural transition (although like childbirth, it can be a hugely different experience from one woman to another).

We need, collectively, to talk about menopause more openly and support one another. Preparation for this stage is paramount. By increasing awareness of perimenopause, I'm hoping that women in their late thirties will also find this book helpful and will be prepared for this transition. I'm also aware that some of you reading this book might have had an early-onset menopause or a medical menopause; if so, this book is for you too, as you navigate, often quite abruptly, these new symptoms. This book is also for trans men, non-binary and gender nonconforming people who I hope will find it helpful too.

I'm very much a realist in my approach. I always focus on consistency rather than perfection, so that sustainable change can occur. There is absolutely no point starting on a journey of change if it's totally unrealistic or unsustainable. This is why many of my takeouts are tiny shifts – even if you only change up the first hour of your day, for example, this will help I promise. My hope is that by the end of this transition we can emerge stronger and wiser than ever.

the problem with modern life

Modern life has had a massive impact on our health. Technology and the fast-paced world we live in have completely untethered us from the natural rhythms of life – including menopause.

DOES THIS SOUND FAMILIAR?

Wake up feeling exhausted...reach for caffeine.

↗   ↘

Feel wired by 11 p.m. and tired, but can't get to sleep.

↑

By 9 p.m. you suddenly feel a clarity of thought you haven't had all day...start doing house admin or answering work emails whilst watching TV.

↑

Eat late.

↑

Head is so frazzled by 5 p.m. that you don't know what to cook, so you snack instead while thinking about what to cook.

Don't feel hungry...skip breakfast.

↓

Spend half the day trying to wake yourself up with caffeine and sugar...and the other half trying to calm yourself down.

↓

No time for a lunch break – eat lunch on the run or in front of a screen.

↓

3 p.m. slump...could fall asleep at your desk, so reach for more caffeine and sugar.

Many of my clients suffer with this back-to-front day – it's a bit like feeling jet-lagged. Our sleep / wake cycle is out of whack because our natural body clock is masked by our turbo-charged modern life: stress, low-nutrient food, stimulants, technology and the artificial light coming from our screens.

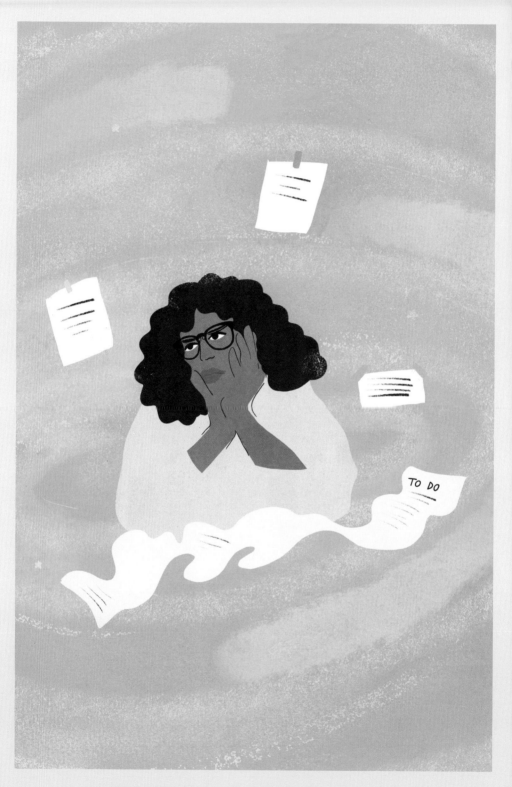

hurried women's syndrome

On top of this omnipresent stress load, we now have to deal with perimenopause. It appears at a time when we're spinning multiple plates in the air and pushing on through our to-do lists like we did in our twenties and thirties. I call it 'hurried women's syndrome'. As women, we have this tendency to look after everyone else except ourselves – even our pets come before us! We don't go to the loo when we should; we don't drink a glass of water or stop to eat; or stop to do any kind of self-care at all. So I feel very excited that you have picked up this book and are committed to helping yourself. The small shifts I'm going to talk about will only take up minimal bandwidth, I promise.

we have it all...but we're exhausted

Stress has such a massive impact on every system in the body, including our hormones. For those of us who have children, we often had them a lot later than previous generations. My mother had me at twenty-three, so I'd left home and was working by the time she hit her late forties. But now women are often navigating perimenopause with the heady mix of young children in the house or, dare I say it, the joy of teenagers. We're also often tied to mortgages based on two incomes, not just one like the baby-boomers enjoyed. Working and being at the top of our game career-wise is another huge strain on our resources, coupled with the way technology has extended the work day and kept our brains busy and disconnected from our body's natural rhythms. Some things do remain the same, though. Women are still more likely to deal with the emotional (unpaid) labour of life: running the house, birthdays, Christmas, social-calendar sorting, connecting with family, dealing with the ecosystem of school and our children's well-being.

menopause in our twenty-first-century world

We work to a male pattern of life. If we choose to have children (19 per cent of us don't[1]), we must peel away from our careers to go on maternity leave and then return having to work even harder to gain promotion versus our male colleagues. The World Economic Forum estimates that we are 267 years away from closing the gender pay gap globally (the UK is ranked 55 out of 153 countries).[2] Menopause is a time when we might be at the top of our career, but suddenly we have to deal with another shift in our body that men simply don't need to address.

The corporate world is still so far behind when it comes to recognizing menopause. Whilst women over 44 represent the fastest-growing demographic in the workplace, some 56 per cent of women experiencing symptoms of menopause had doubted their ability to do their job[3], and 11 per cent had considered resigning.[4] Suddenly we're sitting in a boardroom unable to recall what we were about to say, or we get hot flushes as we're presenting to hundreds of people, or we're completely exhausted from a broken night's sleep. And so much of this is dealt with in silence – nearly half of women have not spoken to anyone at work about their symptoms.[5]

We are also up against medical bias. Staggeringly, menopause is an optional course at some UK medical schools – let's hope this changes soon...menopause affects half the population! 'Psychological weathering' is a term I first heard at a talk by the amazing, Dr Hina J. Shahid. She discussed the triple bias of being a woman, from an ethnic minority and Muslim, and how women of colour have reduced health outcomes because of increased levels of psychological stress, which manifests both physically and mentally.

Karen Arthur,

founder of *Menopause Whilst Black* podcast

No lie, navigating menopause whilst living in a Black woman's body isn't easy. There are no days off. I can't discard my skin when I feel like I need a rest from the shitshow that the world presents us with at times. If you haven't worked it out, I'm talking everyday racism. The daily bombardment of news on the latest murder, missing person, racist headline or thinly disguised public insult. I work hard to counteract this – let's call it what it is – trauma. But all my gratitude lists and affirmations can only go so far. Lasting change lies in the hands of those who aren't heavily invested in caring about Black lives. Menopause loves stress, as we know. So this is why I will always advocate for Black women to take extra-special care of themselves approaching perimenopause and throughout menopause. We must celebrate ourselves when no one else seems to want to. It's why the *Menopause Whilst Black* podcast even exists.

What I will say about menopause is that it has also led me into the best phase of my life. Hands down. Yes, being diagnosed with anxiety and depression and having to leave my teaching career behind couldn't exactly be described as a walk in the park. But I wouldn't have had it any other way. Because now I feel like I care so much less about others' opinions. I'm finally free to do whatever TF I want to do with my own life. Because guess what? It's *my* life!

Listen, menopause can be tough and troubling and worrying, but it can also be liberating and life-affirming, and everything in between. Getting to know myself – what I love and don't love, or how my body reacts to what I consume and how I treat it – has been the gift that keeps on giving, frankly. My body and my boundaries are healthier for it. I wish that for every woman, too.

time to start listening to your body

Your body is changing and you need to stop and listen to it. How often do you override what your body is trying to tell you? We've become quite good at ignoring this – from the advent of our periods, we've learned to keep premenstrual syndrome (PMS) and all other emotions that we feel during our cycles internalized (although I think this is starting to change for our daughters, just as the conversation around menopause is starting to change, too). I work a lot with children in my practice and I'm always in awe of how they naturally listen to their bodies. They listen to those butterflies in the stomach (well, gut really – our stomach is mid-chest, whereas those butterflies are coming from the gut – which is basically our second brain). Sadly, it's a habit we've grown out of as adults. We internalize a lot of the stress that we deal with from society, such as sexism and racism, as well as trying to 'have it all' with a career and / or family. At perimenopause we have to accept that, physically and emotionally, we cannot keep up the pace we lived at in our twenties and thirties. Change can often be an uncomfortable process for those around us – we may start to ruffle some feathers when we start to say no, or to change our boundaries. But I do feel everyone wins in the long term, as we become happier and more contented when we switch patterns of behaviour that haven't been working for us.

Jess Rad,

founder of The WomenHood

It's never been more important to put ourselves first. Having been told that we can 'have it all', women are now desperately trying to 'do it all', which is of course impossible. And the result is chronic stress and burnout. The very concept of rest has become alien to us. Yet what is the impact on our health? What are we modelling to the next generation of girls?

I've discovered that many women want to make changes, but these feel inaccessible amid all the overwhelm. Which is why I advocate just 1 per cent of micro-changes. These tiny, yet remarkable and sustainable alterations to our daily lives really do have the power to change them.

Let's apply this to our most precious resource today – our time. Did you know that 1 per cent of your day is fifteen minutes? How often do you allow yourself that time (screen-free)? Could you gift yourself just 1 per cent of your day, every day? Schedule it. Make it non-negotiable. Then tune in after a week to discover the impact. That to-do list is never going to end. Perhaps it's time to put yourself at the top.

"

TALK TO YOURSELF LIKE YOU WOULD TO SOMEONE YOU LOVE.

BRENÉ BROWN,
RESEARCH PROFESSOR AND AUTHOR

"

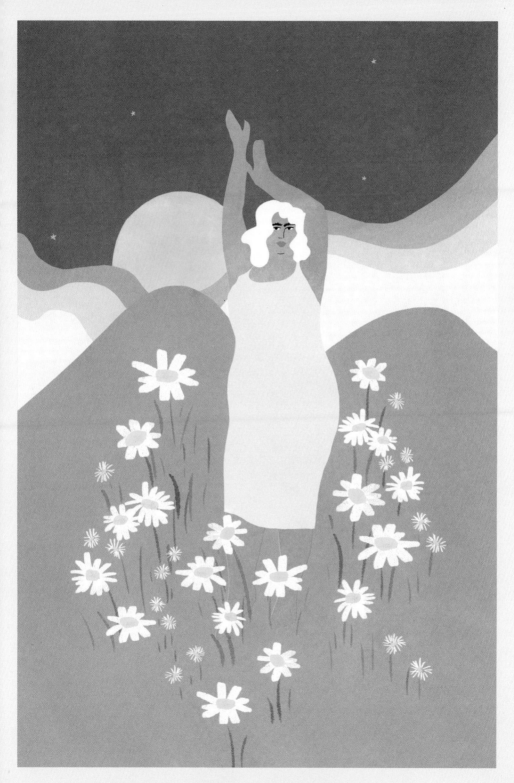

"

THERE IS NO WAY IN
THE WORLD MEN WOULD
PUT UP WITH HOT
FLASHES. I THINK IF
A MAN HAD TWO HOT
FLASHES, THEY WOULD
BLOW THE SUN UP.

WANDA SYKES, COMEDIAN

"

what is going on in my body at perimenopause?

Meno in Greek means 'period' and *pausis* means 'stop'. The term perimenopause is a relatively new one, which describes symptoms that can start happening way before menopause itself. According to the UK's National Health Service (NHS) website, perimenopause usually occurs between the ages of forty-five and fifty-five, the average UK age to reach menopause is fifty-one, and one in 100 women experience menopause before the age of forty. According to NHS guidelines, after a year of no periods you are clinically classified as being past menopause. The Study of Women's Health Across the Nation (SWAN) highlighted that women of colour go through menopause on average two years earlier (at forty-nine) than white women and experience more severe symptoms and sometimes length of symptoms (for instance, hot flushes for ten-plus years). In my experience, women can start to feel changes from as early as their late thirties,[6] but often ignore them until one day they realize things are shifting.

Menopause is a completely natural transition, but it can still be a hugely distressing time physically and emotionally, just as childbirth is a natural event that can still be traumatic – experience of both varies massively from woman to woman. It's a time of fluctuating oestrogen and progesterone that cause these symptoms but, unlike diabetes or hypothyroidism, the body gets used to the lower levels... eventually. We're the only mammals, apart from humpback whales, that live long enough for menopause to take place. The widely accepted anthropological reason why this happens is known as the 'grandparenting hypothesis'. Female whales go through menopause so that they can divert their energy to look after their daughter's offspring, and to spare food resources for their offspring, too.

symptom checklist

Here is a quick symptom checklist – it's interesting to see how far-reaching the roles of oestrogen and progesterone are in the body. Not only do they affect our reproductive system, but they also affect our nervous system (which is why the symptoms aren't just physical, but often psychological, too), our temperature control, our immune system, our skin, our cardiovascular system and our cellular energy. How many of these symptoms are you experiencing? Mark your severity from 0 to 3 – with 3 being as bad as it can be. You can then refer back to this after you have implemented some of my pointers, and hopefully you will see that your scores have moved towards 0...

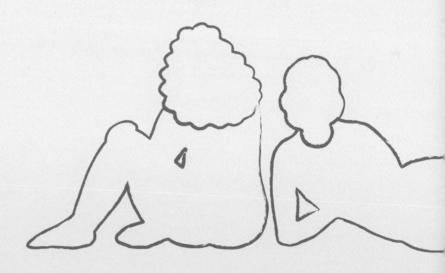

SEVERITY OF SYMPTOMS IN THE LAST WEEK

	0	1	2	3
Aches and pains				
Anxiety / tension				
Bloating / wind / indigestion				
Breast tenderness				
Brittle nails				
Burning mouth				
Coarse hair / hair loss				
Cravings				
Dry, itchy skin				
Facial hair, especially on the chin				
Fatigue				
Foggy head				
Heavier bleeds				
Heightened emotions				
Hot flushes / night sweats				
Increase in allergies				
Insomnia				
Lack of libido				
Low mood				
Low motivation				
Migraines / headaches				
Mood swings				
Muscle weakness				
Nausea				
Palpitations				
Rashes				
Tingling extremities				
Vaginal pain / dryness				
Weight gain (especially around the middle)				

a bit of biochemistry...a quick look at what's going on during our cycle

Remember that perimenopause starts way before your periods stop, hence why the term perimenopause exists (and postmenopause, too, as symptoms can persist after menopause). I'm a big believer in cycle-tracking and there are lots of good apps out there, and for many of us at the start of our perimenopause journey our cycles remain regular, even if our periods have got heavier or lighter. Our cycle effects our body both physically and mentally – we just don't live the same pattern of life that men do. These fluctuations that we experience every month have a massive ripple effect on the whole body – on our energy levels, sleep, digestion, skin, cravings, mental well-being and even our immune system. Tuning into our cycle helps us listen to our body more closely, work out the reasons for low energy, mood swings or sugar cravings so that we can plan ahead and harness our inner power (yes, it is there, I promise) and take time to rest (we tend to ignore this too). Here is a snapshot of what is going on during our cycle.

Starting from the hypothalamus deep inside our brain (often called the conductor of our whole hormone system), gonadotropin-releasing hormone is released, which then stimulates the release of FSH (follicle-stimulating hormone) from the pituitary gland, which in turn encourages the release of oestrogen to stimulate a follicle to be released from the ovaries at the start of our cycle. Then LH (leuteinizing hormone) is released mid-cycle, which stimulates ovulation: the egg is released from the follicle which then goes on to leave a sack-like structure called the corpus luteum, which is the primary site of progesterone synthesis during a regular cycle.

GONADOTROPIC HORMONES

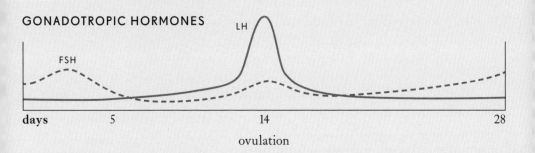

LH

FSH

days   5   14   28

ovulation

OVARIAN HORMONES

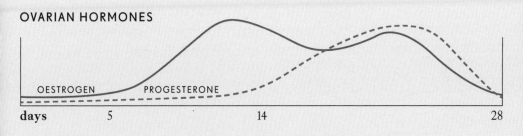

OESTROGEN   PROGESTERONE

days   5   14   28

ONE MENSTRUAL CYCLE

oestrogen

Our body produces oestrogens in three forms: oestrone (E1) is a weaker form of oestrogen and is the predominant oestrogen postmenopause. It is made in peripheral fat tissues and our adrenal glands. Oestradiol (E2) is the predominant form mostly made in the ovaries, and is the most potent in non-pregnant females; and oestriol (E3) is the primary oestrogen of pregnancy, which is largely produced by the placenta. There are receptors all over the body – for more than 300 functions. Oestrogen has far-reaching effects on our bones and skin, insulin sensitivity, brain chemicals like serotonin (our happiness brain-chemical) and heart health…hence the wide-reaching symptoms at perimenopause.

HAS POSITIVE EFFECTS ON: bone health, skin elasticity, heart health, insulin sensitivity, brain chemicals like serotonin and memory.

SIGNS OF EXCESS OESTROGEN: breast cysts,[7] fibroids and history of endometriosis,[8] fat around the middle,[9] heavy periods,[10] low mood[11] and migraines,[12] low sex drive and fatigue.

SIGNS OF LOW OESTROGEN: low libido, memory loss, hot flushes, night sweats, inability to deal with stress, loss of bone density, mood swings, painful sex, vaginal dryness, wrinkly skin and depression.

progesterone

Progesterone helps to prepare the body for conception and pregnancy and is produced after the egg is released from the follicle. The follicle then becomes the corpus luteum, which produces progesterone (this is where imbalances start to happen at perimenopause as sometimes we don't ovulate, meaning no corpus luteum). It's often called the 'everything-will-be-okay hormone', due to its link with GABA, the body's main inhibitory and calming brain chemical, which might explain why the progesterone dip before our menses is when PMS starts to kick in.[13]

HAS POSITIVE EFFECTS ON: bones, breast health, balancing oestrogen, preventing anxiety, PMS and sleep.

SIGNS OF LOW PROGESTERONE: miscarriage, mood swings, irritability, heavy periods, insomnia and anxiety.

testosterone

Testosterone is not just for men! It is made in our ovaries and adrenal glands and in peripheral tissues such as fat cells. At perimenopause we can start to see weight gain around the middle, which is a male (testosterone) pattern of weight storage brought on by declining oestrogen levels. When oestrogen starts to dip, more testosterone is converted to oestrogen by an enzyme called aromatase. Stress increases this enzyme activity which can conversely reduce our testosterone levels.

HAS POSITIVE EFFECTS ON: sex drive, a sense of well-being, memory and vitality which often peaks mid-cycle (when our cycles were regular) when testosterone levels are highest.

SIGNS OF EXCESS TESTOSTERONE: polycystic ovary syndrome, acne, oily skin, excess hair on the face and body.

SIGNS OF LOW TESTOSTERONE: anxiety, depression, low sex drive and low energy.

our cycle

I thought it would be helpful to give a brief overview of our cycle to help us tune into changes that might be occuring. The more we listen to our body, the more we can help to support our symptoms. I recommend cycle tracking to my clients (lots of good apps for this out there, or simply put a P in your calendar). It helps you keep track of where you are in your cycle and how it might be changing.

STAGE ONE: DAYS 1–4, MENSTRUATING

Day 1 is when we start our period. Cycles are usually around twenty-eight days pre-perimenopause, and even in the first part of perimenopause we can have quite regular cycles.

> **HOW WE NEED TO LISTEN TO OUR BODY:**
> Our body is using blood flow as an eliminatory system for the body. Magnesium is a great help here if you suffer from PMS cramping, as it supports all the smooth muscles in our body, of which the uterine muscles are a big part. Up your magnesium-rich foods, as well as using Epsom bath salts around the time of your periods. We need to eat plenty of warming protein-rich foods to help us feel grounded, and iron-rich foods to help boost energy levels and replenish iron stores. We need to rest more at this time, doing mindfulness and meditation and making sure we get enough sleep.

- Menstruation
- Pre-ovulation
- Between ovulation and pre-menstrual
- Pre-menstrual

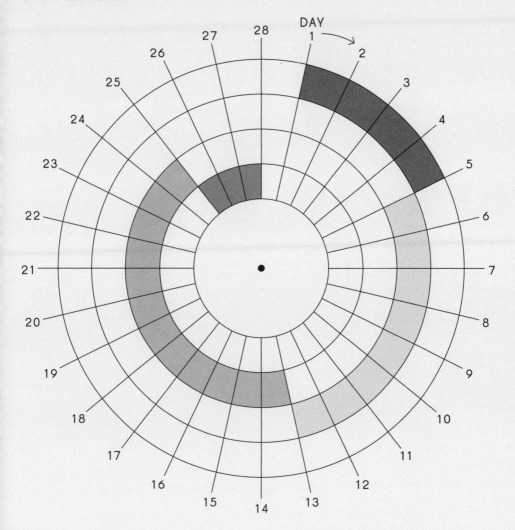

STAGE TWO: DAYS 5–12

The next stage is when oestrogen is starting to rise, and this is often when we feel our strongest, enjoy our exercise and have good mental well-being – oestrogen is a steroid hormone, after all. It helps to build muscle and optimize our bone health, as well as collagen synthesis for our joints and tendons and our skin, too. Our immune system is heightened up to ovulation, because the body is primed to look after our follicle and protect it from bacteria and viruses prior to conception – we are in protection mode.

HOW WE NEED TO LISTEN TO OUR BODY:
It's great to do strength training and cardio at this time of the month and make sure we are supporting our body with plenty of vitamin C, B vitamins, quality protein and omega-3 fats to help build lean muscle, support energy levels and keep inflammation in check. It's fascinating to read about the Chelsea FC Women and how they train according to where they are in their cycle. And at this stage they focus on strength training, but also minimize drills that involve sudden changes in direction, because there was an increased prevalence of ligament tears due to high oestrogen, which increases our ligament flexibility (ready for pregnancy).

STAGE THREE: DAYS 13–25

We get a spike of testosterone at Day 14 to increase libido for conception, which makes us feel strong. Men have ten times the amount of testosterone than we do, which might explain why their libido is often much higher than ours across the entire month. Coinciding with lowering oestrogen, our immune system becomes less 'on guard' mid-cycle to minimize an 'immune attack' from 'foreign invaders' – that is, sperm. This is all designed to help optimize fertilization – which is going on *every single month*. The second half of our cycle is when progesterone is at its highest. If there is a pregnancy, progesterone's role is to maintain it and help the egg embed into the wall of the uterus.

HOW WE NEED TO LISTEN TO OUR BODY:
This can often be a really physically strong time for us too, but then we start to wane as we move closer to premenstrual time. Listen to your body – don't overdo it. Make sure you get outside, to help vitamin-D synthesis through the skin. Plus magnesium, zinc and B6 to help support progesterone production in the second part of the cycle.

STAGE FOUR: DAYS 26–8

Premenstrual time! Oestrogen starts to reduce first, then progesterone – often called the 'PMS hormone' because it dips just before our period, which can lead to PMS symptoms such as low mood and heightened emotions.

HOW WE NEED TO LISTEN TO OUR BODY:

In preparation for menses, this is the time to get one step ahead of our blood sugar. Drops in oestrogen affect our insulin sensitivity, which can lead to carb cravings. Make sure you don't skip meals, and have protein- and nutrient-rich snacks to hand to help keep blood sugar stable, such as trail mix, nuts, seeds, avocado, chicken drumsticks or falafel with hummus. Try to avoid too much refined sugar, caffeine and alcohol (basically liquid sugar), which massively affect the highs and then the lows of insulin. Bloating can also be a PMS symptom, so upping your gut-nourishing food will help here, such as vegetables and fermented foods; avoid lots of gluten, chew your food well and avoid too much sugar and alcohol, which can feed yeasts in the gut.

what is happening to my cycle at perimenopause?

I like to split the phases of perimenopause into two parts.

PERIMENOPAUSE – REGULAR CYCLES

The initial part is when our periods are still regular and changes can be very subtle. We might find that we're more irritable, fatigued, anxious or are experiencing joint pain, PMS and carb cravings.[14] Oestrogen can be hyper-stimulated at this point too which can cause our periods to get heavier.[15] Heart palpitations are often an early symptom – when oestrogen is high, the arteries dilate; and when low, they contract, causing changes in blood pressure that can lead to heartbeat irregularities.[16] These can all be confusing as they're such different symptoms that we don't relate them to our hormones.

PERIMENOPAUSE – IRREGULAR CYCLES

The second phase is when our cycles get shorter or longer – this is why I always advise clients to cycle-track. As our cycles become more sporadic, we might not always ovulate. According to the SWAN study – one of the most comprehensive menopause studies to date – only 23 per cent of women's cycles from a five-year period to menopause were likely to ovulate.[17] This leads to greater dips in oestrogen as well as progesterone. Although oestrogen might still be released (albeit it at lower levels), the majority of progesterone relies on an egg being released. This is why anxiety and intolerance to stress are common perimenopause symptoms. Lower levels of oestrogen can interfere with insulin sensitivity, energy expenditure, inflammation and fat-cell distribution. This is why weight gain, cravings, low energy and weight around the middle are all common symptoms. The change to lower oestrogen and progesterone levels is not a steady one – as oestrogen fluctuates, the hot flushes start to kick in, which are experienced by more than 70 per cent of women.[18]

might you be oestrogen-dominant?

Well-recognized oestrogen-dominant conditions include certain oestrogen-sensitive breast cancers,[19] obesity,[20] endometriosis[21] and fibroids.[22] Additional signs of oestrogen excess prior to perimenopause include: swollen and highly sensitive breasts,[23] anxiety, mood swings, blood-sugar imbalances, heavy periods,[24] brain fog, fatigue, salt and fluid retention, loss of libido, fat around the middle (which produces its own oestrogen[25]), insomnia and PMS.

What's important to note here is that you can remain oestrogen-dominant even in light of reducing levels at perimenopause, and that ovarian hyper-stimulation[26] at the start of perimenopause when our cycles are still regular can also affect this precious ratio between oestrogen and progesterone.[27] So aside from hormone fluctuations, what else causes oestrogen dominance?

* Being overweight correlates with higher oestrogen levels.[28] 'Tummy fat is toxic fat.' Weight around the middle becomes its own endocrine system, converting testosterone to oestrogen, via a process called aromatization, which can increase our oestrogen load.[29] You'd think this would be helpful in light of lowering levels, but the oestrogens produced through aromatization aren't shown to have the same protective effects on the body.[30]
* High stress, lack of sleep and stimulants lead to more emotional eating and high-carb food choices, leading to higher insulin, which then increases weight and excess oestrogen.
* Detoxification issues – we need our liver to be functioning well to break down oestrogen, ready to exit the body.

"

WE KNOW WE MUST
DECIDE WHETHER TO
STAY SMALL, QUIET, AND
UNCOMPLICATED OR
ALLOW OURSELVES TO
GROW AS BIG, LOUD,
AND COMPLEX AS WE
WERE MADE TO BE.

GLENNON DOYLE,
AUTHOR AND ACTIVIST

"

★ Out-of-balance gut bacteria lead to an out-of-balance 'estrobolome' – the interface between the gut and oestrogen balance. Increased beta-glucuronidase enzyme in the gut (especially if you suffer from constipation) can lead to elevated levels of oestrogen being recirculated.[31]

★ We are literally swimming in a sea of oestrogen! We're bombarded by chemicals called xenoestrogens, which are known as 'endocrine disruptors'. They are oestrogen-mimicking chemicals and can be found everywhere – in pesticides and herbicides in our food and water, in plastics, in parabens in skincare products, in exhaust fumes as well as hormones found in our food chain, such as in dairy and meat products.[32]

a note on hormone
replacement therapy

I am very much a complementary, not an alternative, practitioner. When it comes to medications, I am all about informed choice. We are all individual. We all have our own journeys through menopause, and some women are having a torrid time of it – and that's without having to deal with a massive life-load. I have designed this book as a toolkit for whatever your journey might be – and if this includes HRT, the shifts will still be relevant and complementary to you, too. I'm just glad I have this opportunity to discuss the many supports that are available from a nutritional and lifestyle perspective, either with or without HRT.

Dr Olivia Hum,

Menopause specialist

I see HRT as something that can be used to complement any of the other therapies or lifestyle changes. It is one of many ways to make you feel better during menopause – whether that be diet, lifestyle or medication. Anything you can do to help get you through this time and feel better, so that you can get on with your life, is something worth trying.

The fact is that some women feel awful during menopause – they can't sleep, they change personality, they feel anxious, they can't work, their relationships break down. Just because some women sail through by taking a little herbal tea doesn't mean that other women are not really suffering. We need to be sticking together and supporting each other, whatever your route through menopause might be.

We also have this idea that, as women, we have to cope and get on with it. We're busy and we've got a lot on our plates, and we feel we are letting ourselves down if we take medication. The way I see it is that you are lacking in a hormone. If you were low in vitamin D, you would take a supplement without any guilt or shame. For some women the lack of oestrogen is just awful. We need to move away from seeing HRT as a failure to cope, and look at it as one of many possible strategies that can be used to help women through this transition.

PART TWO

The four shifts

"

WHEN WE ARE NO LONGER ABLE TO CHANGE A SITUATION, WE ARE CHALLENGED TO CHANGE OURSELVES.

VIKTOR FRANKL,
NEUROLOGIST AND PSYCHOTHERAPIST

"

INTRODUCTION

My four shifts are designed to help you balance your hormones, support your energy, liver and gut health and kick-start weight loss too. The shifts are designed to help your body gradually get used to lower levels of hormones. We simply do not have to put up with these symptoms just because 'it's our age'.

SHIFT 1:	SHIFT 2:	SHIFT 3:	SHIFT 4:
RESET	CLEANSE	REST	EAT

SHIFT 1: RESET

Shift 1 is all about focusing on our life-load and understanding how stress affects our hormones, especially at perimenopause. We can't walk out of the door and go and live on a desert island (although that would be nice), but we can put ourselves at the top of the self-care list and help our body become more resilient. I'm a big believer that stress can be a positive force, if we can adapt to it.

SO HOW STRESSED ARE YOU?

Do you... [tick the appropriate boxes]

Feel tired all the time? ☐

Have trouble getting up in the morning, even when you go to bed at a reasonable hour? ☐

Feel rundown or overwhelmed? ☐

Have difficulty bouncing back from stress or illness? ☐

Crave salty and sweet snacks? ☐

Have weight gain around the middle? ☐

Feel more awake, alert and energetic after 6 p.m. than you do all day? ☐

Feel irritable a lot of the time? ☐

Have a lower tolerance to stress? ☐

the ancient stress response

Cortisol is our primary stress hormone (along with adrenaline and noradrenaline) and is produced in the adrenal glands (little glands that sit on top of the kidneys), which are hard-wired to the body's 'fight-or-flight' survival response. More than 20,000 years ago this response would have been essential to either fight or run away from a wild animal. The problem is that our body is still wired to be a hunter-gatherer. Unfortunately the body can't tell the difference between running away from a wild animal and sitting at your desk with a coffee getting stressed about spreadsheets – the stress response is the same. Cortisol releases stored blood sugar in our liver and redirects this glucose to the lungs, heart, brain and eyes and away from what it deems unnecessary, such as the digestive, detox, immune and reproductive systems. This is why our periods can stop if we're under a lot of stress (as a protection against pregnancy): the body chooses survival over fertility.

How is cortisol triggered in the body?

1 In response to a stress event

2 By blood-sugar lows

3 By inflammation

> Your brain is designed to keep you alive. It doesn't give a shit about your happiness.
>
> RUBY WAX, COMEDIAN, WRITER AND MENTAL HEALTH CAMPAIGNER

responses to a stress event

Who isn't stressed these days? Stress can be termed as anything that challenges our survival...or even just being busy:

* Physical – trauma, injury, surgery, inflammation, excess exercise
* Chemical – pollution, allergies, blood-sugar imbalance, hormonal imbalance, poor diet, stimulants, drugs, heavy metals
* Emotional: racism, sexism, homophobia, PTSD, lack of love
* Thermal: intense cold or heat
* Infection: illness or serious disease

Elevated cortisol has a negative impact on hormone balance, digestion, detoxification, insulin resistance, obesity, blood-glucose balance, maintenance of lean protein and cognitive function, too. It down-regulates many systems in the body when our body is in fight-or-flight mode and thinks, 'I can't possibly risk getting pregnant now!' or 'I have no time to digest food or detoxify – I have to focus on surviving above everything else.' It also has a massive effect on our sleep by completing mucking up our sleep / wake cycle, called our diurnal rhythm (for more on this, see page 78).

What's important to know at perimenopause is that our adrenal glands produce a twelve-times weaker form of oestrogen called oestrone, which is primarily made there, and progesterone, too. As oestrogen from the ovaries declines, we become more reliant on this weaker form and on an adrenal source of progesterone. The adrenals should be our ovary back-ups so we need to be mindful that stress (survival) trumps sex hormones!

self-care for the beginning of the day

1. Drink a warm cup of water with a slice of lemon on waking. It helps to stimulate your liver and adds a little vitamin C.

2. Do fasted exercise when you have the time (exercise before you eat anything or drink caffeine).

3. Take your supplements (have them out by the kettle).

4. Enjoy a high-protein breakfast to boost your metabolism and help reduce the need for so much caffeine; eggs any which way; a green smoothie using more veg than fruit; low-sugar granola with almond or coconut yogurt; Bircher with oat milk, ground linseed, grated ginger and cinnamon and berries; scrambled tofu; avocado with grilled mushrooms and tomatoes.

5. Enjoy your caffeine only with your breakfast.

6. Take time to eat your breakfast – enjoy and look forward to it!

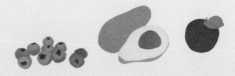

SMALL SHIFTS: SELF-CARE

Aside from food, these other tools might help too:

- Laughter (it stimulates endorphins,
  our feel-good chemicals)

- Building a sense of gratitude for small things

- Cultivating healthy social relationships and
  parking less helpful ones

- Spending time in nature – I love the
  Japanese concept of 'forest bathing'

- Fun and play – I think many
  of us don't give ourselves
  time to have fun anymore

- Movement

- Dance – kitchen disco!

- Active rest – don't feel guilty
  for stopping and staring out the
  window for a bit!

the problem with caffeine

Caffeine basically puts us into fight-or-flight mode. It elevates cortisol and adrenaline levels, both at rest and in periods of stress. So even though your day might not be stressful, your caffeine will be making you more on edge – which is why you can get that jangly feeling if you've had too much. Don't get me wrong: I get a huge amount of joy from my coffee, but I enjoy one or two cups a day only at breakfast (I have recently switched to decaf, which has massively helped my stress levels and afternoon energy).

Nourishing our adrenal glands is so important at midlife to help us become more resilient to stress, and to support the weaker form of oestrogen and progesterone production as our ovaries start to quieten. Only drink caffeine with breakfast (or replace with a decaf or herbal tea). Food helps to reduce caffeine's metabolic effect, too.

The adrenals love:
* Vitamin C: green leafy vegetables, parsley, citrus fruits, peppers, kiwis, dark berries.
* B5: egg yolk, broccoli, fish, shellfish, organic yogurt, legumes.
* B6: broccoli, Brussels sprouts, cabbage, cauliflower, kale, nuts, pumpkin, spinach.
* Protein: bone broth, eggs, brown rice, oily fish, tofu, tempeh, pulses, quinoa.
* Magnesium: black beans, pumpkin, sunflower and sesame seeds, green leafy vegetables, almonds, spinach, Swiss chard, Epsom bath salts.
* Blood-sugar balancing helps to reduce the need for cortisol (see page 48–53).
* Adaptogens help to blunt the stress response: maca, turmeric, Rhodiola rosea, liquorice (tea) and ashwagandha.

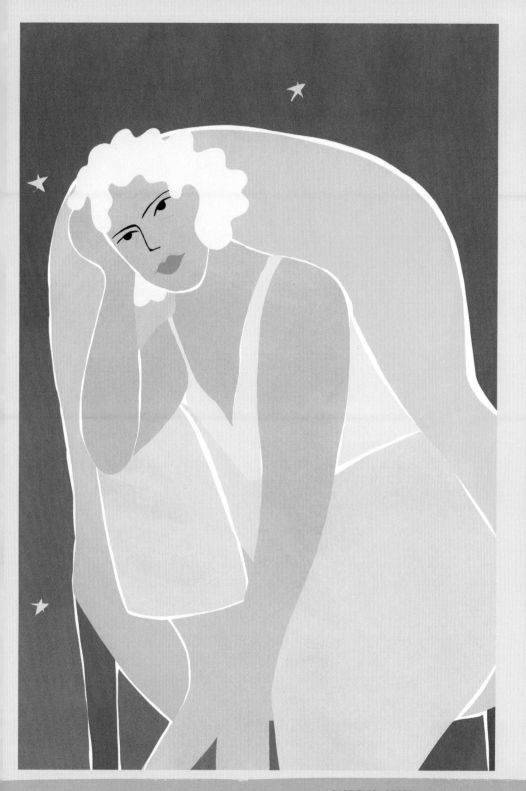

blood-sugar balancing

As I mentioned, I can't do anything about your external stress (I am sorry about that), but I can help your body need cortisol less by keeping blood sugar balanced. Oestrogen helps to keep blood sugar balanced, which is why cravings and imbalances can become worse at perimenopause as oestrogen dips.[33]

Do you suffer from any of these symptoms?

* Feel shaky, clammy or faint before eating?
* Get that need to eat now feeling?
* Get hangry?
* Feel like a different person after eating?
* Wake often at night?
* Find it hard to go without food for more than two hours?
* Eat lots of refined carbs?
* Are susceptible to cravings and emotional eating?
* Crave sugar, pasta or bread?
* Get sleepy in the afternoon?

If you answered yes to any of these questions, then your blood-sugar balance is probably in need of some support.

The brain's preferred fuel is glucose, so the brain keeps it within a tight range. The illustration opposite shows that range lying between the grey lines. When we eat refined sugar, our blood sugar spikes and stimulates insulin production. Insulin is produced in our pancreas and its role is to bring down blood sugar in the blood and store it as fat in our fat cells. It is our primary storage hormone. Often after this high we can get a low of blood sugar. If you suffer from low mood, irritability, anxiety or emotional eating, these blood-sugar lows will exacerbate such issues. Lows of blood sugar are coupled with a sense of guilt and strong cravings to refuel the brain – and this is when emotional eating can really come into play. A sugar low stimulates the stress hormones cortisol and adrenaline to bring the blood sugar back up again. The more our blood sugar is out of whack, the greater the need for stress hormones!

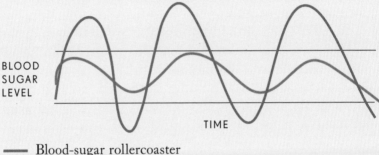

BLOOD SUGAR LEVEL

TIME

—— Blood-sugar rollercoaster
—— Normal blood sugar

I liken sugar to pouring petrol onto a fire – the flames burn really bright and kick out a lot of heat (blood-sugar high), which can give us a sense of energy; but after this short spike the flames become even smaller than they were before (blood-sugar crashes). Putting protein and good fats on the fire I liken to coal – although the flames don't burn as brightly, more heat is produced and they burn for longer (which gives us a drip feed of energy, and heat equates to satiety, so fewer cravings). Don't be fooled into thinking that fake sugar is better. I'd actually rather that you had real sugar. Aspartame, xylitol and stevia are often more than 180 times sweeter than sugar and can trick the body into thinking it's getting something sweet, but in fact nothing arrives, which creates more of a craving.

emotional eating

Staying one step ahead of cravings will help you feel more on an even keel and less likely to eat emotionally. We have forgotten *why* we eat. It's rare for many of us to feel hunger. Instead we are often ruled by 'emotional hunger', which is often unsatisfied by food, so we feel the need to eat more. The neurochemical dopamine in our prefrontal cortex is all about reward, and cravings are dominated by the dopamine reward system. It's often called the 'dopamine pleasure trap'. Unfortunately, highly processed food causes a rise in dopamine and this reward-seeking behaviour. We 'eat our emotions' rather than eating because we're hungry. The Japanese call it *'kuchisabishii'* that literally means 'lonely mouth' or 'longing to put something in one's mouth'. Here are the physical and psychological differences:

* **Physical hunger:** builds gradually; grumbles in the stomach are due to the hormone ghrelin, which tells us we could do with some food; it is satisfied by eating; occurs after time has passed since your last meal.

* **Emotional hunger:** often not caused by being physically hungry, but by boredom, reward seeking, anxiety, sadness, fear, loneliness or commiseration, for example, if you've had a bad day.

So how do we fix this? In order to rewire our feelings of emotional hunger it's important to stay one step ahead of those emotional rollercoasters where feelings of guilt, shame or self-criticism are high. Sugar control is very important to rewire our hunger cues, along with adding more micronutrients, protein and fats into our diet, so that we feel more grounded and satisfied. This helps to 'crowd out' the cravings. Always question *why* you're eating. The more you do this, the more you will start to find contentment in the fact that sometimes you might really want that cake and learn to be mindful and really enjoy it, with no sense of guilt attached.

food swaps

DESIRED FOOD/DRINK	→	SWAPPED FOOD/DRINK
Chocolate	→	Dark raw chocolate, dark-chocolate-covered Brazil nuts
3 p.m. biscuits	→	Trail mix, miso soup, falafel, hummus, almond butter on a corn cake, low-sugar almond or organic soya yogurt with some low-sugar granola
Cup of tea/coffee	→	Herbal teas like fresh mint (which doesn't work so well with biscuits, helping to remove the association/reward cue), fresh juice, water
Crisps	→	Toasted chickpeas or teriyaki seeds, olives
Wine	→	Sparkling mineral water with a slice of lemon, sliced ginger and cinnamon in a cup of hot water, fresh mint tea, chamomile tea

Chains of habit are too light to be felt until they are too heavy to be broken.

WARREN BUFFETT, BUSINESSMAN AND PHILANTHROPIST

perimenopause and insulin sensitivity

As our oestrogen levels start to dip, this can make us less sensitive to insulin,[34] which means that the cell receptors are basically putting down their shutters and saying, 'Nope, we don't need any more glucose', which means higher blood-sugar levels and more fat storage. This then impacts on weight gain and food intake which is why it is so much harder for us to lose weight at perimenopause and why balancing our blood sugar is so important.

the worry waist

This is a classic sign of too much cortisol. It is also due to declining oestrogen levels – the change to abdominal fat is a much more male (testosterone) pattern of weight gain. Suddenly we start to gain weight around the middle or get a 'muffin top'. Our waist begins to disappear. And the problem with these central-weight fat cells is that they are not inert, like fat stores on the bottom, hips and thighs. Unfortunately this central weight interferes with our hormones as it starts to convert testosterone stored in these central fat cells to oestrogen. These oestrogens produced from testosterone via a process called aromatization aren't shown to have the same protective effects on the body. Central fat cells start to produce inflammatory cytokines and, as cortisol is our natural anti-inflammatory hormone, this has the effect of stimulating the adrenals to make more cortisol to deal with the inflammation, too. The more stressed we are, the worse we sleep; and the worse we sleep, the less resilient to stress we are during the day, which leads to more stimulants and low-nutrient food, which in turn makes our sleep worse. For more on menopause weight loss, see the Troubleshooting section on pages 148–51.

SMALL SHIFTS: BLOOD-SUGAR CONTROL

- Fast for twelve to fourteen hours overnight and micro-fast between main meals.

- Don't skip breakfast – eating earlier in the evening will help you feel hungrier on waking. Breakfast time is when you need the energy.

- Eat protein and beneficial fats at every meal to stay one step ahead of carb cravings.

- Only drink caffeine with breakfast. Have herbal teas for the rest of the day or water instead of tea and coffee to help break the association with biscuits.

- Remember that alcohol is liquid sugar.

- Ultra-processed chocolate bars have harnessed fat and sugar, which never occur together in nature, therefore causing our reward centre to go into hyperdrive. Opt for raw cacao chocolate instead – it is so bitter you won't need as much.

- Identify the emotional eating cues – the most powerful cues happen around the same time and place every day.

- Change the routine – actively interrupt the routine and replace it with a new one.

- Change the reward – the reward positively reinforces the routine and etches the habit on the brain. Opt for non-food rewards such as a hot bath with Epsom salts, being in nature, alone time or time with friends.

inflammation nation!

Inflammation is essential in the body in order to alert you that there is a problem. For example, if you sprain your ankle, the pain, swelling and redness (inflammation) will alert you not to walk on it, so that the body can repair it. Declining oestrogen levels can make us more inflamed because oestrogen is one of our natural anti-inflammatory steroid hormones – one of the reasons why we can start to suffer with aches and pains (see more on this in the Troubleshooting section on page 109). There is even new research describing perimenopause as a 'pro-inflammatory phase'[35] due to these declining oestrogen levels. Cortisol is an important anti-inflammatory hormone, so the more inflammation we have, the more stress hormone we need! Many of us are inflamed even before we enter perimenopause, so an important shift is to help reduce our inflammatory load. There is so much that can be done to help put out those flames of inflammation through diet and lifestyle.

Do you...

Get bloated?
Suffer from a nasal drip?
Suffer with skin conditions such as rosacea, psoriasis or eczema?
Get aches and pains (pain = inflammation)?
Get a foggy head?
Carry weight around the middle?
Eat lots of pro-inflammatory foods, such as processed food, sugar, alcohol, meat and dairy products?

OMEGA-3 AND -6

Both omega 3 (alpha-linolenic acid) and omega-6 (linoleic acid) are essential fatty acids (EFAs) needed in our diet.

- Omega-6-rich foods include meat, dairy products and vegetable oils (not olive oil). They provide a form of omega-6 called arachidonic acid, which has the pro-inflammatory properties needed when we are injured, feverish, for muscle repair, healthy brain function and blood clotting.

- There is another kind of omega-6 called gamma linolenic acid, which has anti-inflammatory actions: from evening primrose, hemp and borage oil.

- Omega-3 foods include oily fish such as salmon, sardines, trout and mackerel, and a vegan source from algae (usually in supplement form), which are all sources of EPA and DHA, which provide an anti-inflammatory action. Linseeds/flaxseeds, linseed/flaxseed oil, hemp oil and nuts such as walnuts are vegan sources of omega 3 and need to be converted from alpha-linolenic acid to EPA and DHA.

The problem with our modern-day diet is that the optimum ratio of 3:1 omega-6 to omega-3 is now much greater – some would put it at 20:1.[36] So we have too many ON inflammation switches and not enough OFF ones. Meaning that we have a skew towards more pro-inflammatory EFAs. In addition to this, our diet is high in processed foods (made with bad fats), additives, sugar, alcohol, caffeine and gluten,[37] which all have pro-inflammatory effects on the body.

SMALL SHIFTS: ANTI-INFLAMMATORY ACTIONS

- Reduce pro-inflammatory omega-6 foods, including meat, dairy, refined vegetable oils (use olive oil instead) and processed foods.

- Up your omega-3 foods. It's the omega-3 anti-inflammatory foods that we often need more of vs. the pro-inflammatory omega-6 foods.

- Reduce alcohol (see page 64), refined sugar and gluten (see page 67), which all have a pro-inflammatory effect.

- Address gut inflammation (see page 66).

- Address fat around the middle, which can add to the inflammatory load (see the Troubleshooting section on pages 148–51).

- Up your phytoestrogens (see page 91).

I've discovered that this is your moment to reinvent yourself after years of focusing on the needs of everyone else.

OPRAH WINFREY

SHIFT 2: CLEANSE

Cleansing is incredibly important to help reset our hormones. It helps to support our detoxification pathways in the liver, to balance our gut microbiome, to keep inflammation in check and make sure we eliminate all those toxins and excess hormones. Our gut microbiome is a like our bacterial garden! Home to trillions of microorganisms which rely on plenty of diverse fibre (our gut bugs love variety!) to keep this vital ecology in balance. Our gut microbiota, or gut bugs, eat what we eat.

It also helps to reduce those xenoestrogens from the food chain. I've included my 14-Day Cleanse for those that want to kick-start new habits and weight loss, too.

how to eat

However great your diet, if it's not being digested properly then it's a waste of time. We are what we digest! New areas of research into chrono-nutrition demonstrate that eating earlier in the day has wide-reaching metabolic benefits.[38] The problem for most of us is that we eat our main meal at the end of the day when we don't need the energy – we need that at breakfast. Eating later in the evening is also likely to affect how well the food is digested.[39] However, I totally get that eating in the evening often coincides with friends and family time – I'm a big believer in food as community, and the importance of eating with loved ones (however monosyllabic our children or partners might be); this is still an important time of the day.

low digestive function

So here are some classic signs and symptoms of low digestive function:

1. Don't feel hungry on waking.
2. Don't feel hungry until mid-morning or maybe not until lunchtime.
3. Feel full quickly after eating.
4. Get a pain in the right-hand side.
5. Feel nauseous after eating fatty food.
6. Suffer with reflux or heartburn.
7. Feel bloated after eating.

Digestion actually starts in the mouth – our saliva glands excrete carbohydrate-digestive enzymes, and our chewing is essential to help masticate our food so that it's easier to break down in the stomach and beyond. But so many of us inhale our food, without really chewing much at all. Here's how I help clients to slow down their eating using the raisin test:

* Get yourself two raisins or sultanas.
* Eat one like you'd usually do.
* Then take the other one and hold it up and look at it: look at the ridges, feel how squishy it is, smell it, then place it in your mouth and savour the way it tastes. Then chew it slowly – aim for ten times (it might disappear before then, but give it a go).
* This is a prime example of how 'mindful eating' can slow down your eating, if you're a speedy eater.

SMALL SHIFTS: HOW TO EAT MINDFULLY

- Don't eat in front of a screen – you're more likely to eat without even realizing it, so that after your meal has finished you need more.

- Eat slowly – by eating with friends or family, and put your knife and fork down between each mouthful if you tend to 'inhale' your food.

- Chew each mouthful ten times.

- Avoid drinking large quantities of water with meals, as it can put out your stomach-acid fire.

- Don't eat when stressed.

- Don't eat when on the move.

- Wait twenty minutes before going for seconds, as this gives the food time to reach the gut to signal that you no longer have hunger.

- Are you hungry or are you actually thirsty?

- Eat an earlier evening meal so that you feel hungrier on waking to give your body the energy when it needs it – at the start of the day.

- Avoid going to bed soon after eating.

eating like our ancestors did

Our body hasn't changed in 20,000-plus years. It is in serious need of an upgrade. So while we wait a few thousand years for that to happen, I'd recommend mimicking our ancestors when it comes to eating habits, as much as possible. They would definitely have had to expend energy to feed themselves…but now we simply have to make it to the kitchen cupboard. We are constantly eating – and often pre-empting hunger, too. When was the last time you allowed yourself to feel really hungry?

The easiest and simplest way to mimic our ancestors is to have periods of fasting in between meals of three to four hours, and twelve to fourteen hours overnight. Doing exercise while fasting first thing in the morning or between meals also helps to fat burn and leads to lean muscle mass and better blood-sugar handling. Remember that as soon as we eat, insulin spikes which puts us into storage mode.

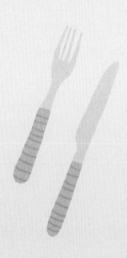

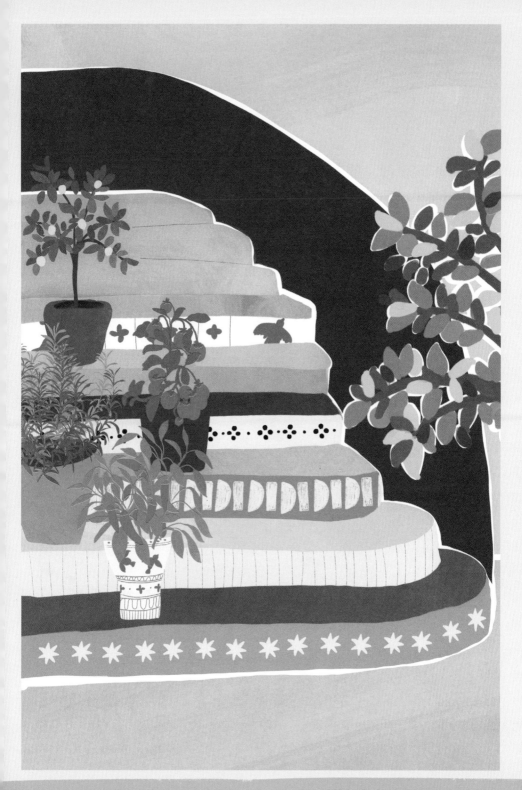

liver TLC

Our liver is the major multitasking organ of the body. It has more than 500 functions, which include being our detox powerhouse, digesting fat and getting rid of excess cholesterol, converting fat to glucose (vital for energy production), clearing the blood of infections (50 per cent of our lymph is made in the liver), clearing excess oestrogen and other hormones, converting the thyroid hormone T4 into the more active T3, and storing the fat-soluble vitamins (A, K, E and D) – and this is why eating liver is such a great source of vitamin A (although not something I shall be recommending!). The liver is so important that it takes a staggering 30 per cent of our blood flow every minute. It can spring-clean itself and can indeed regenerate, but it needs proper nourishment, which is often lacking in our modern-day diet as it struggles to deal with toxins from medication, alcohol, sugar, fructose, caffeine, the xenoestrogens in pesticides and plastics, the parabens in skincare products, the hormones and antibiotics found in the animal food chain, plus air pollution.

Naturopathically, the liver is regarded as the organ of anger, judgement and mood. It doesn't have any nerve endings, so it's hard for us to tell if it's overworked and in pain. Here are some common signs and symptoms of low liver function...

Do you...
1. Feel sick after fatty food?
2. Suffer from hives or itchy skin?
3. Feel hungover super-fast after alcohol?
4. Get terrible hangovers?
5. Have a sensitivity to chemical smells or perfumes?
6. Suffer from anger and intolerance to stress?

When it comes to our hormones, the liver is crucial for hormone-balancing. Sex hormone-binding globulin (SHBG) is produced here, which keeps our hormones in check. It is also needed to detoxify oestrogen into weaker forms ready for excretion via the gut. This is why whenever I'm helping women to balance their hormones, the liver is an incredibly important organ to support.

The liver can spring-clean itself – the body will always be detoxifying – but the beauty of optimizing nutrition is that we can flood the body with micronutrients so that it can basically do its job better. We also want the liver to not have to deal with so many toxins, so a two-pronged attack is required.

SMALL SHIFTS: THINGS TO TAKE OFF YOUR PLATE

- Reduce your intake of fried foods, high-fat foods and fructose in the form of pasteurized fruit juices (not freshly made juices – they can stay).

- Check on your skincare products – are they adding to your toxic burden?

- Avoid too much caffeine, and only have it with food to lessen the effects.

the problem with alcohol

Alcohol is simply not very helpful to us at perimenopause. It's liquid sugar, for a start, which can cause those blood-sugar dips; it has a massive effect on restorative sleep; hangovers lead to eating more refined carbs and caffeine the next day; and it can cause gut inflammation and uses up our zinc stores.

With alcohol, I like the focus to be on excellent quality and drinking less of it. It's the same premise I have when eating meat or chocolate and when drinking coffee: high-quality, mindful consumption, but less volume. I'm also done with hangovers.

Do you feel pressure to drink in social situations? In the UK if you say you're not drinking, people think either you're an alcoholic, pregnant or a party pooper. My tip is to accept the drink – the chances are they'll not be watching when you actually drink it, so you can happily hold the glass all evening. That gets rid of having to explain what's going on at the start of the evening. I'm always conscious that if someone I know says 'No, thanks' to a drink, then I respect that decision and offer them something non-alcoholic. Aside from the fact that I don't have a problem with people not drinking, if they have a drink problem, then saying no probably took a lot of strength and courage so labouring the point is the worse thing you can do.

SMALL SHIFTS: LIVER FOODS

- The liver loves brassicas – they contain a compound called indole-3-carbinol, which helps the liver detoxify oestrogens more efficiently. So try to eat them daily: broccoli, cabbage, cauliflower, kale, Brussels sprouts.

- Bitter foods help to retract the gall bladder and allow bile to flow freely (which helps to digest fats and get rid of excess cholesterol). So eat bitter leaves such as artichoke, chicory and rocket, plus chamomile, peppermint, liquorice, dandelion and burdock tea.

- Try making green smoothies with: dark berries, cucumber, greens of your choice, almond butter, ginger, avocado and water.

- Turmeric (curcumin) and ginger are also big liver tonics, as is a hot water with lemon on waking – always part of the first hour of my morning self-care routine. You can finely slice ginger and add it to hot water, and keep adding to it through the day, although if you are getting hot flushes, turmeric and ginger can be quite heating, so better to opt for the lemon instead.

- Keep yourself hydrated.

- Selenium helps support detoxification and is found in: Brazil nuts, chicken, eggs, halibut, liver, sardines, spinach and turkey.

gut TLC

The gut is our biggest defence against the outside world, other than the skin, and is where we absorb most of our nutrients. Its microbiota – the bugs in our gut – house more than 100 trillion microbes, weighing around 2 kg/4½ lb. What we eat has a huge effect on our microbiota.[40] The gut is also where two-thirds of the immune system is housed and it's home to the largest number of nerve endings outside the central nervous system – it's basically a brain.[41] The largest amount of our 'happiness neurotransmitter', serotonin, is made here, too. The manifestation of long-term stress can cause irritable bowel syndrome (IBS), anxiety and depression, often with constipation, because we hold so much emotion in our gut.

So is your gut in balance?
* Do you go for a bowel movement every day?
* Or is it rabbit droppings?
* Do you suffer from constipation?
* Do you have an urgency to go?
* Do you not feel properly evacuated?
* Do you suffer from bloating, wind, colic or churning?
* Do you get IBS-like symptoms?
* Do you suffer from recurrent thrush, athlete's foot, fungus on the skin or under the nails or a white tongue?
* Do you have more than two bowel movements a day?

> ❝ All disease stems from the gut. ❞
>
> **HIPPOCRATES**

If you answered yes to any of the above, then you're probably in need of some gut TLC. Ideally there should be an eighteen-hour transit time from mouth to butt. If it's too quick then it is likely that the nutrients aren't being absorbed properly, which can fuel fatigue. If you're having days of not going, or frequent rabbit droppings, then this can affect your hormone balance.

the problem with constipation and our hormones

According to the NHS website, constipation is classified as not going for at least three days in one week, your stools are dry or lumpy or hard and there is pain or straining. Rabbit droppings can be a sign of impacted stools, where only the outer bits are coming off. Gut support is always part of what I call my oestrogen-clearing programme to help ensure that we go once a day, ideally on waking, and we should feel fully evacuated after going. The problem with constipation is that it can lead to oestrogen not being eliminated through the stools and getting reabsorbed via the liver back into the body, causing higher oestrogen levels. This is down to the gut's ability to moderate oestrogen in the body, called the estrobolome, but constipation can upset this balance.

the problem with gluten

Gluten is Latin for 'glue' and has been shown to increase intestinal permeability or a 'leaky gut'.[42] We don't need to be coeliac for gluten to cause us problems – there is much research on what is now known as 'non-coeliac gluten sensitivity'.[43] Gluten simply isn't very helpful, and for many of us we have too much of it – tea and toast or gluten-rich cereals for breakfast, followed by a sandwich for lunch and then pasta for dinner. I recommend that clients opt for gluten-free where possible (gluten-free pasta has come a long way in the past few years) and then you can naturally move towards more nutrient-dense options. For many of us, we can tolerate gluten, so if you do eat it, then buy the best, freshest bread, cake, biscuit or pasta you can afford, eat it mindfully and enjoy it.

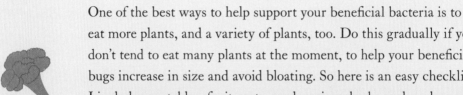

the plant-variety tracker

One of the best ways to help support your beneficial bacteria is to eat more plants, and a variety of plants, too. Do this gradually if you don't tend to eat many plants at the moment, to help your beneficial bugs increase in size and avoid bloating. So here is an easy checklist. I include vegetables, fruit, nuts, seeds, spices, herbs, pulses, legumes, grains (ideally gluten-free). Aim to start with a goal of thirty unique plants a week and work up to forty-plus and then fifty-plus.

WEEK 1		
1.	11.	21.
2.	12.	22.
3.	13.	23.
4.	14.	24.
5.	15.	25.
6.	16.	26.
7.	17.	27.
8.	18.	28.
9.	19.	29.
10.	20.	30.

WEEK 2

1. _____	9. _____	17. _____	25. _____	33. _____
2. _____	10. _____	18. _____	26. _____	34. _____
3. _____	11. _____	19. _____	27. _____	35. _____
4. _____	12. _____	20. _____	28. _____	36. _____
5. _____	13. _____	21. _____	29. _____	37. _____
6. _____	14. _____	22. _____	30. _____	38. _____
7. _____	15. _____	23. _____	31. _____	39. _____
8. _____	16. _____	24. _____	32. _____	40. _____

WEEK 3

1. _____	11. _____	21. _____	31. _____	41. _____
2. _____	12. _____	22. _____	32. _____	42. _____
3. _____	13. _____	23. _____	33. _____	43. _____
4. _____	14. _____	24. _____	34. _____	44. _____
5. _____	15. _____	25. _____	35. _____	45. _____
6. _____	16. _____	26. _____	36. _____	46. _____
7. _____	17. _____	27. _____	37. _____	47. _____
8. _____	18. _____	28. _____	38. _____	48. _____
9. _____	19. _____	29. _____	39. _____	49. _____
10. _____	20. _____	30. _____	40. _____	50. _____

SMALL SHIFTS: FEEDING THE GUT

• Up your variety of unique plants – starting with thirty-plus per week.

• Eat fermented foods, if tolerated – sauerkraut, kefir, miso, kombucha, kimchi.

• Drink 1.5–2 litres/2¾–3½ pints of water daily.

• Too much protein from red meat, dairy products and gluten can contribute to constipation. Increase vegetable sources of protein instead (pulses, lentils, rice, quinoa and soya products).

• Avoid too much refined sugar, which feeds yeasts.

• Go gluten-free, or avoid gluten as much as possible, especially if you are constipated.

• Make sure all pulses are soaked, cooked, fermented or sprouted to reduce lectins, which can cause wind.

- Magnesium is needed for smooth muscle contractions – the gut is one long, smooth muscle.

- Fresh pineapple and papaya are sources of the protein-digesting enzymes bromelain and papain.

- Eat omega-3-rich foods: linseed/flaxseed, pumpkin and sesame seeds, walnuts and oily fish.

- Eat stewed apples for their pectin.

- Oats are rich in beta-glucans (soluble fibre), which provides food for gut bacteria, and fibre.

- Ground linseed/flaxseed helps to bulk up stools.

- If you've had antibiotics recently, have a course of high-potency probiotics.

- Jerusalem artichokes, chicory, asparagus, leeks – a source of prebiotics to support healthy bacterial balance.

my 14-day cleanse

Here is my gentle 'you can still function in the real world' 14-Day Cleanse – the shopping list even includes chocolate! Once you reach Day 14, you have finished. So technically the Cleanse is really thirteen days… For maximum benefit it's important to slowly re-introduce the foods not included in this Cleanse, although you should feel energized and not want to swing back to old habits. You can track six health parameters. Assess them at the start, midway and at the end of the Cleanse, and you should notice an improvement. For each of the following, rate how you feel on a scale of 0–6 – with 6 being as good as it can be, and 0 being as bad as it can be.

TRACKING HEALTH PARAMETERS

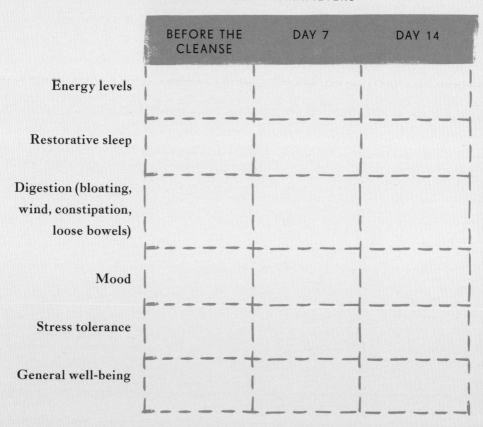

	BEFORE THE CLEANSE	DAY 7	DAY 14
Energy levels			
Restorative sleep			
Digestion (bloating, wind, constipation, loose bowels)			
Mood			
Stress tolerance			
General well-being			

HERE ARE SOME GENERAL CLEANSE POINTERS:

* Opt for two weeks when you don't have much going on. Self-care and allowing yourself to go slowly are very important here.

* If you have a regular cycle, then aim to cleanse during the front half, when sugar cravings are low and energy is higher.

* Try to coincide the Cleanse with some breathwork, yoga or meditation at the start and end of the day to help keep the focus on listening to your body.

* If you get light-headed or excessively fatigued, it may be a sign of low blood sugar, so keep an apple or pear handy to have if low blood sugar strikes.

* During Days 3–4 you may want to curtail some of your more strenuous activities, as you may experience a decrease in energy. This won't last long – you will then start to feel more energy than you ever knew you had.

* You may get aggravations, especially if you normally have a lot of caffeine, sugar or wheat. Headaches are common, as is feeling 'fluey'. These are often manifestations of toxins on the move, but usually after a day or two these sensations go and you are left with more energy.

* Keep up your exercise, but go easy on yourself – this is when yoga or meditation will be helpful.

* Avoid eating the same foods every day. Eat a variety of foods, and rotate the meals.

* Aim for consistency– don't beat yourself up if you have a less-than-perfect day.

MINDFUL EATING

Throughout the Cleanse take time to eat whenever you can. Eating when stressed or on the go really doesn't help our digestive function, as the stress hormone cortisol down-regulates our digestive system because the body is in fight-or-flight mode, not rest-and-digest mode. Enjoy your food time, eat slowly and aim to chew ten times.

WHAT TO AVOID WHILE ON THE CLEANSE

* Gluten (wheat, rye, barley, spelt)
* Dairy products
* Caffeine (you can try to come off one cup at a time prior to starting the Cleanse, to avoid headaches)
* Alcohol (fresh herbal tea and a little dark raw chocolate at alcohol pinch-points helps, such as in the evening)
* Meat, fish and eggs
* All refined sugars
* Hydrogenated fats
* Processed foods
* Processed-fat spreads
* Chips and other fried vegetables
* Artificial colourings
* Flavourings and sweeteners

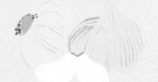

WHAT TO EAT IN ABUNDANCE

* Vegetables!
* Eat dark leafy greens every day (kale, watercress, parsley, rocket, etc.)
* Eat cruciferous vegetables daily to support the liver (broccoli, cabbage, cauliflower, etc.)
* Have onion or garlic daily
* Protein from quinoa, brown rice, tofu, falafel, hummus, pulses, legumes
* Antioxidant-rich foods: any brightly coloured fruit and veg (including green and white), such as berries, cherries, parsley,

squash, carrots, spring greens, spinach, figs, pomegranate, plums

* Fruit for sweetness, or almond, coconut or plain yogurt and sweeten with a little honey, cinnamon or blueberries; dark chocolate, as detailed in the shopping list on pages 76–7
* Herbal teas instead of caffeine: fresh mint, sliced ginger with lemon, lemon and a stick of cinnamon, (avoid rooibos).
* Keep hydrated – aim for eight glasses of water daily (be careful not to down a large pint of water at mealtimes, as this might put out your stomach-acid fire)
* Drink a warm cup of water with a slice of lemon on waking
* Exercise/move daily – but be mindful of resting if you start to get a drop in energy or headaches; this will pass

Some hormone-balancing extras:
* Phytoestrogens are balancing to both excess and low oestrogen states: soya (tofu, tempeh, miso, natto, edamame beans), chickpeas, lentils, peas, ground linseed/flaxseed, sesame seeds, cashews, kale, broccoli, brussel sprouts, carrots, cabbage, cauliflower, peppers, cherries, garlic, apples, apricots, soybean sprouts, alfalfa, split peas, pinto beans and red clover
* Note the importance of the brassica family (see page 92): indole-3-carbinol is a precursor to diindolylmethane (DIM) and is found in cruciferous vegetables: broccoli, cauliflower, kale, cabbage, sprouts

A NOTE ON SNACKING

The Cleanse programme is full of beneficial protein, fat, antioxidants and gentle fibre, which help curb emotional eating as you get used to less refined sugar and fewer processed foods. You will notice a shift in your energy levels as you come off the blood-sugar rollercoaster. Try to fast overnight to give your digestive system a break. Many of us eat most of our food at the end of the day, when it's more likely to be laid down as fat. I'd also recommend mini-fasts in between meals, but if you find this too hard, there are snack options.

SHOPPING LIST

The shopping list will help you keep one step ahead of cravings, but it is only a guide – see what works for you. I recommend purchasing some glass Tupperware for leftovers, to be used for lunches. Batch cooking is a great way to save time at the stove and cash, too. Below are some foods that I class as store-cupboard essentials, but there's no need to get them all. I'm hoping that the new eating practices you experience will stay with you way beyond the fourteen days.

* **Pre-packed foods for on the go:** organic nut butters, falafels, pulses and brown rice, vegan kimchi (without fish sauce) and sauerkraut, almond yogurt, soya yogurt, coconut yogurt, hummus, tamari-flavoured seed mixes, dark raw chocolate

* **Fermented foods, if tolerated:** coconut kefir, sauerkraut, vegan kimchi, miso; make sure they are as fresh as possible and not pasteurized as this can affect their fermentation quality

* **Seasoning:** using herbs and spices instead of salt: bay leaf, mint, dill, marjoram, caraway seeds, fenugreek, nutmeg, chives, garlic, cinnamon, cardamom, cloves, allspice, curry leaves, lemongrass, za'atar, paprika and smoked paprika, saffron, fresh basil, oregano, keffir lime leaves, ginger, turmeric, tarragon, curry powder, mustard seeds, nigella seeds, fennel seeds, five spice, cumin, garam masala, coriander, black pepper, cayenne pepper, nutritional yeast

* **Pastes and sauces:** gluten-free soya sauce, tamari, porcini mushroom paste, harissa paste, red and white miso paste

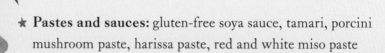

* **Nuts and seeds:** sunflower, linseed, pumpkin and sesame seeds; Brazil nuts, cashews, hazelnuts, almonds, walnuts; avoid peanuts

* **Teas:** Liquorice, if you are very stressed; fresh ginger if you have aches and pains

- **Vegetables and herbs:** carrots, celery, squash, sweet potatoes, green beans, broccoli, cauliflower, peas, mushrooms, cabbage, avocado, beetroot, kale, chard, asparagus, pak choi, Brussels sprouts, spinach, chives, leeks, shallots, parsley, dried porcini mushrooms, dried shiitake mushrooms, dried daikon

- **Grains** – avoiding all gluten grains: brown, wild and white rice (brown is preferable), corn, oats, quinoa, polenta, buckwheat, millet, amaranth, rice noodles, sweet-potato noodles (find these in any Chinese supermarket)

- **Legumes and pulses:** tinned or soaked chickpeas, black beans, kidney beans, butter beans, haricot beans, flageolet beans, red and brown lentils

- **Dairy alternatives:** oat milk, almond milk, coconut oil instead of butter, almond or coconut yogurt

- **Soya products (organic where possible):** tofu, tempeh, edamame beans, miso, organic soya yogurt

- **Sweeteners:** agave syrup, raw honey

- **Dressings:** extra-virgin olive oil with lemon, raw cold-pressed nut and seed oils (do not use for cooking – these are for salad dressings), such as fresh linseed/flaxseed oil

- **Fruit:** apples, pears, melon, figs, berries (can be purchased frozen and used for smoothies); maximum: two portions a day

- **Fats and oils:** linseed/flaxseed oil and hemp oil (never heat it), coconut oil (can be heated), best for baking as a good alternative to butter; nut butter (cashew or almond)

linseed oil

SHIFT 3: REST

Dips in both oestrogen and progesterone affect how well we sleep at perimenopause. Progesterone is linked to a calming neurochemcial in the brain called GABA which helps increase alpha waves so we can sleep. When progesterone drops, this affects GABA.[44] Oestrogen is linked to serotonin which is a precursor to melatonin – the sleep hormone.[45] Hot flushes, night sweats (see pages 126–8) aches and pains (see pages 109–10) and anxiety (see pages 113–15) are also reasons why our sleep deteriorates even further at perimenopause.

Some sleep stats:
* We spend one-third of our life sleeping.
* In an average lifetime we will spend around six years dreaming – more than 2,000 days.
* Approximately 20 million people in the UK struggle with insomnia and other sleep problems.
* On average we now go to bed and wake up two hours later than a generation ago.
* We're getting 20 per cent less sleep per night on average than we were forty years ago.
* Artificial light is listed as a probable carcinogen by the World Health Organization.

And unfortunately at perimenopause the sleep stats get even worse:[46]
* Perimenopausal women aged forty to fifty-nine are more likely to sleep for less than seven hours (56 per cent) than post-menopausal (40.5 per cent) and pre-menopausal women (32.5 per cent).
* Post-menopausal women are more likely than pre-menopausal women to have trouble falling asleep (27.1 per cent compared to 16.8 per cent, respectively) and staying asleep (35.9 per cent compared to 23.7 per cent).

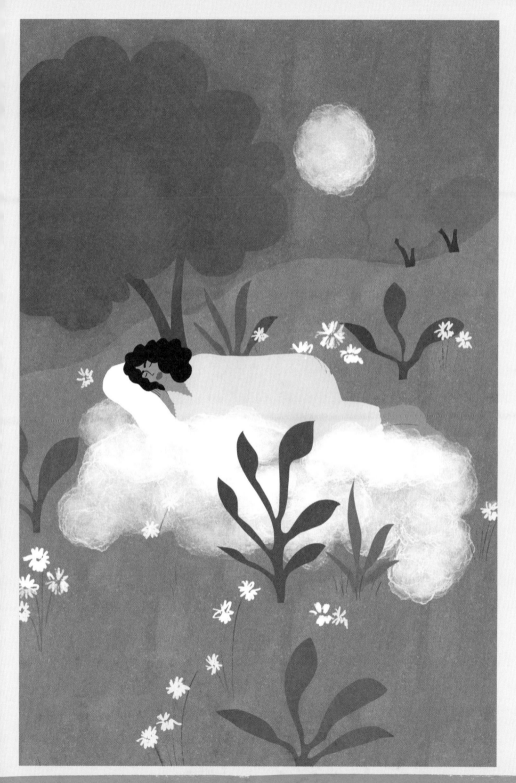

why do we sleep?

* Sleep is an anabolic state during which the body replenishes its energy storage, regenerates tissues and produces proteins.
* Sleep makes us think better.
* During the day brain cells build connections with other parts of the brain as a result of new experiences. During sleep the most important of these connections are strengthened and the unimportant ones are pruned.
* Cerebral fluid increases during sleep to help clean up the brain and clear it of waste – a bit like a dishwasher.
* Studies have shown a reduction in amyloid plaque during sleep cycles.

The main sleep issues I see in my clinic

* Do you have difficulty falling asleep?
* Do you have problems staying asleep?
* Do you wake up feeling mentally and physically exhausted?

tomorrow starts today!

We've become so untethered from our natural body clock that many of our other functions have also become out of whack. We used to get up as the sun rose and rest at nightfall; we used to eat following the path of the sun. But light in our homes and other stimulants have stopped this from happening. If the body thinks it's still daytime, then this is when we get our second wind, cortisol is kept high and melatonin is kept low. Our ancient body clock – our circadian rhythm – controls many other processes in the body aside from our sleep / wake cycle:

* Immune function
* Digestion function is highest at the start of the day, and lowest in the evening.
* Cortisol is highest on waking, to help us feel refreshed and should gradually dip to its lowest at 10 p.m. to aid restful sleep and melatonin production.
* Our blood pressure is lowest at night and slowly gets higher on waking.[47]

sleep foods specific to perimenopause and beyond:

Phytoestrogens to help with serotonin/melatonin production: soya (tofu, tempeh, miso, natto, edamame beans), chickpeas, lentils, peas, ground linseed/flaxseed, sesame seeds, cashews, kale, broccoli, Brussels sprouts, carrots, cabbage, cauliflower, peppers, cherries, garlic, apples, apricots, soybean sprouts, alfalfa, split peas, pinto beans and red clover. Magnesium, zinc and B6-rich foods to help with progesterone / GABA production: broccoli, black beans, cabbage, avocado, kale, nuts, pumpkin seeds, prawns and tofu.

difficulty falling asleep

Have you spent the whole day trying to keep yourself awake, only to find that you get that second wind in the early evening? I have so many clients who could literally start their day at 10 p.m. If you suffer from this, then you are very much not alone. This is a classic sign that your circadian rhythm is out of sync.

SMALL SHIFTS: WIRED-AND-TIRED TROUBLESHOOTING

- Avoid too many stimulants in the day: tea and coffee, sugar, chocolate, alcohol.
- Blood-sugar balancing (see page 48–53).
- Ditch screens in your bedroom, and come off them altogether an hour before bed (use special glasses to help dull the stimulating blue light from screens).
- Magnesium is known as nature's tranquilliser, and magnesium-rich foods include: black beans, avocado, pumpkin, sunflower and sesame seeds, almonds, spinach, Swiss chard; and don't forget Epsom bath salts.
- The glycine-rich proteins found in skin and gelatinous cuts of meat can improve sleep quality. Bone broth!
- Avoid bacon, cheese, chocolate, cured meats, sausages, fermented foods, yeast and wine close to bedtime. These foods all contain tyramine, which increases the release of the brain stimulant noradrenaline.
- Herbal teas are helpful prior to bedtime: chamomile, valerian, lavender, lemon balm and passionflower.
- Don't eat too late – heat from the digestion can affect sleep.
- Don't exercise too late at night.

problems staying asleep

Many of us get to sleep okay, but wake up in the night, usually at the same time. Survival is making us wake up! Being dead to the world for 8 hours wasn't good for our safety 20,000-plus years ago, so if you can go back to sleep after waking, this is perfectly normal.

According to Traditional Chinese Medicine, our organs are busy at certain times of the day, which makes sense to me as we would be exhausted if they were all super-busy at the same time: 2–3 a.m. is when our liver is the busiest, and this is often the time when my clients wake up. It's interesting that when I work with clients with a sleep monitor, I can immediately see the difference in restorative sleep when they don't drink alcohol. Many clients drink in the evening to help themselves sleep, but alcohol can interfere with the alpha and delta brain waves needed for restorative sleep.

SMALL SHIFTS: STAYING ASLEEP TROUBLESHOOTING

- Monitor the change in your sleep when you've drunk alcohol versus non-drinking days.
- If you've had alcohol at dinner or during the evening, prior to going to bed have a small snack (such as some nut butter on a rice cake, a couple of spoonfuls of coconut or soya yogurt or a few olives), as this may help to lessen any blood-sugar lows during the night that may wake you.[48]
- Tryptophan-rich foods to help your sleep include: bananas, figs, dates, nut butter, oat cakes, kiwis, tart cherry juice.
- Have a journal by your bed for any busy thoughts when you wake up.
- See Insomnia on page 129.

tired on waking

So many of my clients wake up feeling exhausted. Hopefully this book and its small shifts will help. The problem is that because we feel so tired, we reach for stimulants all morning to try and wake ourselves up, which then affects how we sleep and so the cycle continues. But there are things you can do to break this catch-22, and they all happen in the first hour or so of your day. The ripple effect across the rest of the day will help you to sleep better.

SMALL SHIFTS: TIRED-ON-WAKING TROUBLESHOOTING

- Invest in a sunrise alarm clock, which gradually lights up to help boost your wakefulness.
- Drink some water on waking to help rehydrate you.
- And lemon and hot water to wake up the liver.
- Start your day with a protein-based breakfast.
- Only have caffeine with your breakfast – herbal teas for the rest of the day.
- Take a ninety-second break when you feel dips in energy – your brain will love it.
- Eat earlier at night, to help you feel hungrier on waking, ready to take on nutrients to help energize you.

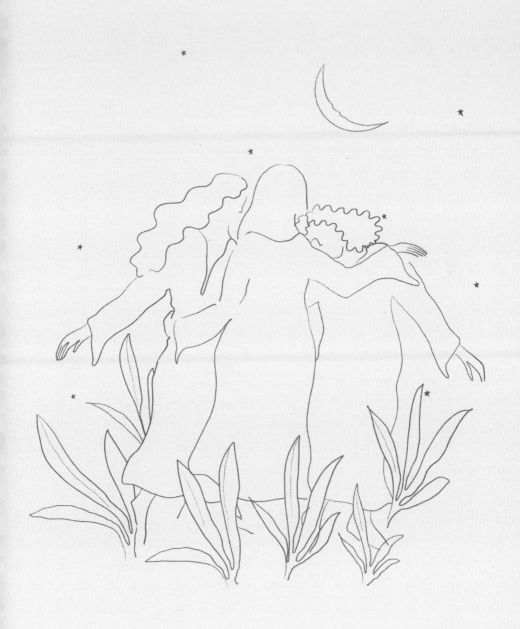

SMALL SHIFTS: SOUND SLEEP RITUALS

- Get some vitamin D during the day – being outside more has been shown to increase melatonin production, our sleep hormone.

- Aim for the same bedtime every day – routine is helpful here.

- Buy yourself an alarm clock to replace your phone.

- Use the bedroom only for sleep and sex – not for watching TV, using the computer, etc.

- Cool the bedroom – keep the window open.

- Don't go to bed too late or you may get your second wind.

- Don't nap during the day, if this is not something you usually do.

- Exercise in the late afternoon, but not right before bedtime.

SHIFT 4: EAT

I think a lot about what I'm going to cook… One of my biggest daily joys is eating. I'm a big believer in the power of food as love and as community, and I often talk to my clients about eating as close to nature as possible, to connect us to the ebb and flow of the seasons.

The focus of this part of the book is to move us from energy-dense to nutrient-dense foods – foods that give us a massive micronutrient hit of minerals, vitamins, omega-3 and -6 essential fatty acids and phytonutrients. So often we're low in these sparkplugs, as I like to call them – the car might have enough petrol (macronutrients: protein, fat and carbohydrates), but it won't go without those tiny sparkplugs (the micronutrients). They're essential for thousands of chemical reactions that are happening in our body every second. Lower levels of micronutrients mean that our body won't run as efficiently as it should do. We need a thereaputic diet at perimenopause, not a 'balanced' one!

Although we have an abundance of food, we're often starved of nutrition. My clients often don't have an unhealthy diet – there's not a mountain of fried food or takeaways, or sugary drinks or sweets; it's just very low in 'sparkplugs'. So I thought it would be useful for you at this point to keep a three-day food diary. No marks out of ten, I promise! I always find it is a good exercise for my clients to see in black and white what they are consuming. As you move through the book you can start to make the small shifts that I recommend, to help move your food choices from energy-dense to more nutrient-dense options.

"

ONE CANNOT
THINK WELL, LOVE
WELL, SLEEP WELL,
IF ONE HAS NOT
DINED WELL.

VIRGINIA WOOLF,
WRITER

"

THREE-DAY FOOD DIARY

	WEEKDAY 1	WEEKDAY 2	WEEKEND 1
Example – breakfast	*Cup of tea with cow's milk + slice of brown toast with jam*	*2 x tea, skipped breakfast*	*2 x tea with scrambled eggs on toast*
Breakfast			
Lunch			
Dinner			
Snacks			
Alcohol			
Caffeine			

my therapeutic foods for menopause plate

40% vegetables (whole, not processed), including fermented vegetables such as sauerkraut and kimchi and brassicas such as broccoli

25% protein-rich food – oily fish, white fish, eggs, organic meat, legumes, pulses, tofu, tempeh, edamame beans, nuts, seeds, quinoa

10% grains (ideally gluten-free), such as brown rice, quinoa, oats

10% healthy fats – nuts, seeds, olive oil, coconut oil, avocados, kefir, full-fat yogurt

10% fruit (whole, not processed): eat a rainbow of colours

5% herbs and spices – make your own pesto, chimichurri sauce or salsa verde to up your plant variety

General pointers:
* Hydration – all our body ever needs to drink is water.
* Avoid too much processed food.
* Avoid too much refined sugar.
* Only have caffeine with food.

phytoestrogens

Phytoestrogens are structurally very similar to oestradiol.[49] However, they are not oestrogen and exert a much weaker effect on the oestrogen receptor sites of cells. The clever thing about phytoestrogens is that they combat fluctuating oestrogen symptoms.[50] They have been shown to reduce oxidative stress[51] and, as such, improve cardio-disease risk,[52] help lumbar-spine bone density and to alleviate hot flushes.[53] There is ongoing research into their role as protection against the risk of breast cancer, due to their oestrogen-modulating properties.[54][55][56] However, I should note that there remains a lack of consensus in the scientific literature.

* Soya foods like tofu, tempeh, soya yogurt, miso, natto, edamame beans are used for soy isoflavones, which are also found in chickpeas, lentils and peas.

* Only eat cooked or fermented soya products, because raw soya has more lectins, which can affect the uptake of iodine in the thyroid. Lectins are deactivated by soaking, cooking and fermentation.

* Lignans are another family of phytoestrogens – linseed/flaxseed is the highest source then sesame seeds (tahini!), cashews, kale, broccoli, Brussels sprouts, carrots, cabbage, cauliflower, peppers, cherries, garlic, apples, apricots.

* Coumestans are another group and include soybean sprouts, alfalfa, split peas, pinto beans and red clover.

* Use sage – as a herb, in tea or as a supplement and red clover – in tea or supplements.

* You do need lactic acid in the gut to absorb phytoestrogens from these kinds of foods: probiotics, kefir, sauerkraut, kimchi, miso, kombucha.

soya and the thyroid

Only eat cooked or fermented soya, as raw soya
contains more lectins – a protein found largely
in pulses and grains. Lectins are seen as toxic, but
soaking, cooking and fermenting them can reduce
their toxic element. Research into fermenting soya beans
reduced their lectin content by 95 per cent[57] and sprouting by 59
per cent.[58] There have been suggestions that the lectins found in
soya can affect the uptake of iodine in the thyroid, although a risk
assessment conducted by the European Food Safety Authority
(EFSA) in 2015 found there was no risk between soya isoflavones
and thyroid function.[59] Plus a large systematic review of eighteen
randomized controlled trials on soya and thyroid also concluded
there was no effect.[60]

the importance of the brassica family

The indole-3-carbinol found in brassicas is the precursor to
diindolylmethane (DIM), which is found in cruciferous vegetables
(broccoli, cauliflower, cabbage, sprouts) and has been shown to
reduce the conversion of oestrogen into 16-hydroxyestrogen, which
is linked to cellular proliferation, and instead to promote the
conversion into 2-hydroxyestrogen, which is a weaker, and far
less proliferative form.[61] Raw brassicas, plus soya and peanuts,
are known as 'goitrogens', which may inhibit thyroid hormone
production by decreasing iodine uptake; however, research is based
on their raw form and seems only to be an issue if iodine is low. So
eat brassicas cooked, and if you don't have an iodine issue,
then the huge benefits you get from eating them far outweigh
any possible negatives.[62]

protein

Protein is the building block of the body. It is incredibly important at midlife as it helps to sustain energy levels, fuel detoxification and support lean muscle mass. There are 9 essential proteins (amino acids) that we must get from our diet: histidine, isoleucine, leucine, lysine, methionine, phenylalanine, threonine, tryptophan and valine. We don't store protein in the body like we do fat and glucose, so a steady flow of it is needed with every meal from high-quality sources such as grass-fed meat, organic poultry, eggs, oily fish, white fish, legumes, pulses, nuts, seeds, tofu; even vegetables have some protein, too.

fats

Fat is our friend. Saturated fat gives us greater energy gram for gram than carbohydrates which is why it makes us feel satisfied for longer. This is why I prefer full-fat versions when buying yogurts for example. Low-fat yogurts might be low-fat but they often have a lot of sugar in them (which converts to fat in the body) that creates more hunger soon after eating, as they don't satisfy us as much! Then we come to essential fatty acids. These are the omega 3 and 6 fats which are not made in the body, we must get them from our food. They're essential for our mental well-being, nervous system, cell membranes, skin, cardiovascular health and hormone-signalling. Omega-3 fats are abundant in oily fish, nuts and seeds and seed oils such as linseed/flaxseed oil. Omega-6 comes from meat, dairy, vegetable oils, borage or evening primrose oil. Olive oil, coconut oil and butter are good fats to use for cooking.

carbohydrates

We still need carbs, but the complex ones – the ones that are slower to release their sugar, versus the quick-releasing refined carbs variety.

✱ **Complex carbs:** squash, sweet potatoes, oats, asparagus, broccoli, cauliflower, artichokes, beetroot, Brussels sprouts, cabbage, carrots, celery, cucumbers, aubergine, courgettes, rhubarb, peppers, garlic, lettuce, spinach, mushrooms, onions, turnips, watercress

✱ **Refined carbs:** white rice, pasta, potatoes, white bread, cakes, biscuits, pastries, ultra-processed foods, many breakfast cereals, sweetened fizzy drinks

fibre

As you will see repeated again and again in this book, green leafy vegetables are so helpful, so eat your greens. They are stacked full of vitamins and minerals, plus all-important fibre. The recommended daily allowance (RDA) for fibre in the UK was almost doubled in 2015; it went from 18 g/½ oz to 30 g/1 oz. And many of us only just get enough. The benefit of getting fibre from plants (not grains such as gluten) is that they help to feed the beneficial bugs in our gut and massage it on the way down. It's also essential if you have high cholesterol and as part of weight loss – fibre increases the stretch receptors of our stomach to help us feel more satisfied.

vitamins

Water-soluble vitamins are carried by water –
they're more unstable than fat-soluble vitamins.
Unlike fat-soluble vitamins, they are more likely to leak out with
water released after chopping or cooking. When cutting veg and it
discolours this is a sign of vitamin C leaving the building! Always
steam rather than boil to minimize losses. Never buy pre-chopped
veg and consume or cook quickly after chopping to retain these
vital nutrients.

* B vitamins – or memory vitamins – help with low energy,
  depression and anxiety. They can be found in eggs, cereals,
  brown rice, fish, chicken, asparagus and dark green vegetables.

* B6 is super-important at perimenopause and throughout our
  entire hormonal journey, which is why it's going first. It is
  needed for progesterone support – get it from broccoli, Brussels
  sprouts, cabbage, cauliflower, kale, nuts, pumpkin, spinach and
  wholegrains.

* B3 for blood-sugar balancing – from meat, fish, eggs and green leafy
  vegetables.

* B5 for adrenal support – from egg yolk, broccoli, fish, shellfish,
  organic yogurt, legumes, mushrooms, avocado and sweet
  potatoes.

* B9 folate for healthy red blood cells, DNA synthesis and protein
  metabolism – from egg yolk, dried beans, lentils, split peas, soya
  bean, almonds, sweet potato, spinach, beetroot, sprouts, broccoli,
  cauliflower, kale, cabbage, pak choi and asparagus.

* B12 for energy, healthy oxygen supply and the nervous system – from beef, chicken, eggs and fish, particularly trout and salmon.

* Vitamin C is a powerful antioxidant that helps fight off free radicals. Plus it supports brain health and collagen synthesis as we age, and mental agility, too – from citrus fruits, parsley, maca powder and green leafy vegetables.

Fat-soluble vitamins need fats to digest them, and are stored well in the body.

* Vitamin A – via beta carotene which converts to vitamin A in the body, for example, from green leafy vegetables; orange-coloured fruit and veg; legumes, wholegrains; and vitamin A directly from oily fish, organic full fat yogurt and egg yolk.

* Antioxidant vitamin E – from nuts, seeds, eggs, wheatgerm and green leafy vegetables – to help with proper functioning of vitamin A.

* Vitamin D, the sunshine vitamin, is needed for mental well-being, calcium balance, bones, the gut and our immune system. The best food source is oily-fish skin. Best of all is making vitamin D from sunshine (using an appropriate SPF factor) or taking a supplement: make sure it is the D3 form, and emulsified, which will help it digest better.

* Vitamin K is good for blood clotting and bone density – from dark-green leafy vegetables, especially kale, broccoli, chard, sprouts, spinach and parsley.

useful minerals

* Magnesium is regarded as nature's tranquillizer and is needed for 300-plus functions in the body, including aiding sleep and energy production; plus helping to alleviate constipation, PMS cramping and migraines. Magnesium-rich foods include wholegrain rice, pumpkin, sunflower and sesame seeds, almonds, cashews, oats, brown rice, avocado, black-eyed beans, spinach and Swiss chard. And don't forget Epsom bath salts.

* Zinc-rich foods help anxiety, obsessive-compulsive disorder, acne, stomach acid production, the immune system, hormone synthesis, our skin, taste and smell – get zinc from lean beef, pumpkin seeds, crustaceans, sesame seeds and dark raw chocolate.

* Calcium is calming (hence the old-fashioned way we'd be given a glass of milk before bed), but we don't need to live near a dairy herd to survive. If you think about what a cow eats all day to produce calcium-rich milk, it's grass. So leafy greens are a great source, and not only do they give us calcium, but they also give us loads of other minerals that are needed for strong bones. For more on this, see the Osteoporosis section on pages 141–3. Other sources, aside from dairy products, are almonds, sardine bones, anything green and leafy, broccoli, cabbage and tofu.

* Iron provides energy, and iron from meat is easiest to absorb – but if you are a non meat eater you just need to make sure you have vegan sources in abundance – get it from darker cuts of chicken, lean beef, green leafy vegetables (especially spinach), quinoa, brown rice, pumpkin seeds and tofu.

* Selenium is needed for thyroid support and liver detoxification – from Brazil nuts, sardines, prawns, salmon, beef, turkey, chicken, eggs and brown rice.

phytonutrients

These tiny compounds are not on any government RDA list, but are hugely important for health. They help plants fend off viruses, funghi and bacteria. Some common phytonutrients include:

* Resveratrol – in red wine, grapes, blueberries and cranberries

* Flavonoids, include quercetin (nature's antihistamine), flavones and anthocyanins – in citrus fruits, parsley, kale, onions, cherries, berries, apples, ginger and chocolate

* Lycopene – in tomatoes and watermelon

* Ellagic acid – in raspberries, pomegranate and berries

* Indole-3-carbinol – in brassicas

* Genistein – in soya

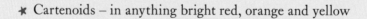

* Lignans – in ground linseed

* Cartenoids – in anything bright red, orange and yellow

* Curcuminoids – in turmeric

the perimenopause store-cupboard

* Phytoestrogens: soya (tofu, tempeh, miso, natto, edamame beans), chickpeas, lentils, peas, ground linseed/flaxseed, sesame seeds, cashews, kale, broccoli, Brussels sprouts, carrots, cabbage, cauliflower, peppers, cherries, garlic, apples, apricots, soybean sprouts, alfalfa, split peas, pinto beans and red clover

* Fish and seafood: omega-3-rich oily fish (see page 55), white fish, plus prawns and all other crustaceans

* Adaptogens: turmeric, ginger, maca, liquorice, ashwagandha, rhodiola

* Fruit: cherries, blueberries, pomegranates, plums, lemon, mango

* Vegetables: beetroot, avocados, brassicas, fennel, garlic and green leafy vegetables

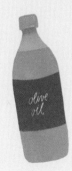

* Eggs

* Wholegrains: brown rice, wild rice, quinoa, oats

* Nuts and seeds: pumpkin seeds, sesame seeds, walnuts, Brazil nuts, almonds, linseeds/flaxseeds

* Oils: butter, coconut oil, olive oil, linseed/flaxseed oil (not recommended for heating/cooking)

* Meat: poultry, lean beef

* Fermented foods: kefir, kimchi, sauerkraut, miso

* Dark chocolate (raw, non-dairy such as coconut)

* Teas: sage, green tea, peppermint, fennel, ginger root, chamomile, cinnamon, liquorice, red clover

* Nervine herbs help with mood swings – chamomile, hops, celery, valerian and lavender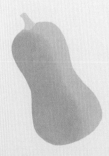

* Cooling foods – tofu, chicken, eggs, apples, pears, lemon, sage tea, millet, cucumber, celery, peppermint tea, green juices

Perimenopause and menopause should be treated as rites of passage. If not celebrated, then at least accepted and acknowledged and honoured.

GILLIAN ANDERSON, ACTOR

supplements

Not all supplements are made equal. And this often give supplements
a bad rap. My first rule of thumb is never to buy supplements from
your supermarket – they are likely to be lower-potency or not in
the right format (which is often cheaper to make). A classic example
of this is magnesium oxide versus the more bioavailable forms of
magnesium citrate, glycinate and sulphate (the last being the format
of Epsom bath salts). It is usually much better to buy supplements
from your local independent health-food store, as the people who
work there generally have a good knowledge of different brands and
the options for your particular health needs.

The focus in my clinic is always on food first, but supplements
can help to break catch-22s like digestive under-function, or speed
up healing (I'm all for channelling a little Barbara Cartland, who
famously took more than sixty supplements a day!).

Here are the top brands that I use regularly in my practice – the
brackets relate to companies that specialize in certain areas: Allergy
Research Group, A. Vogel, Bare Biology (omega-3), BioCare,
Bio-Kult, Bionutri, Biotics, Cytoplan, Floradix, Higher Nature,
Invivo (probiotics), Lamberts, the Linseed Farm (linseed oil and
linseed meal), Naturya (organic-powdered foods, such as maca, acai,
spirulina and chlorella), Nutrigold, Renew Life (probiotics), Sun
Chlorella, Unbeelievable Health, Westlab (Epsom salts) and
Wild Nutrition.

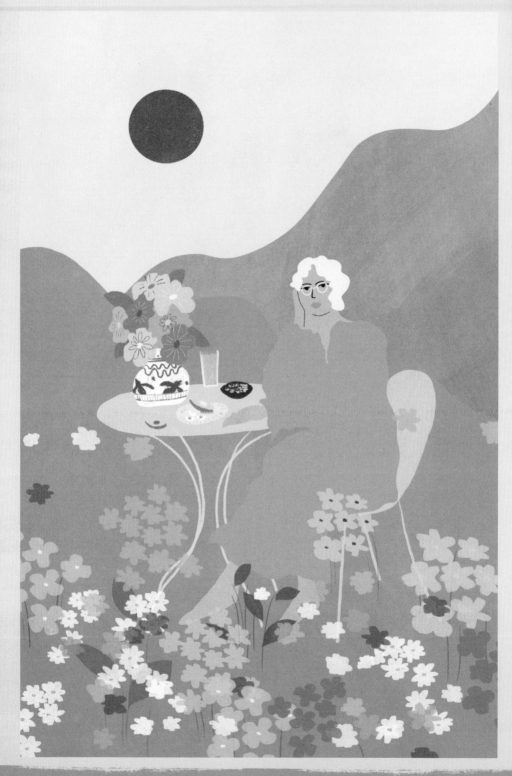

eat with the path of the sun – the importance of breakfast

If there is one thing you action from this book, eating breakfast would probably be my number-one shift. Because we don't feel hungry on waking, we may simply reach for tea or coffee and a slice of toast, because we feel we ought to eat something. Breakfast is so important because:

* It give us energy for the day ahead.
* It helps us curb caffeine (and then we sleep better).
* We don't need to snack so much.

I used to live in Vietnam and China and have always thought how intelligent their eating practices are, as they eat the same savoury, nutrient-rich food for breakfast, lunch and dinner. Only we in the West think a piece of burnt gluten (toast) with jam, or a sugary or glutenous breakfast cereal coupled with skimmed cow's milk (not even full fat), plus pasteurized fruit juice (giving us only fruit sugar), is the way forward – no wonder we often get a sugar crash at 10.30 a.m.

SMALL SHIFTS: MY TOP WEEKDAY BREAKFASTS

1. Eggs! Scrambled or poached eggs go nicely on a bed of spinach that naturally wilts, or with grilled tomatoes.

2. Full-fat almond yogurt/organic soya yogurt/coconut yogurt with low-sugar granola, plus berries and two tablespoons of ground linseed/flaxseed.

3. Porridge with almond or oat milk, cinnamon or ground cardamom and either stewed apples or cut-up pear, or sliced figs with two tablespoons of ground linseed/flaxseed and a little grated ginger.

4. Bircher muesli using rolled oats, with cinnamon, two heaped tablespoons of ground linseed/flaxseed, figs, blueberries or whatever is in season, plus grated ginger and some grated turmeric for extra warmth. Add a dollop of almond or coconut yogurt, if extra protein is required.

5. Avocado sliced on some sourdough or gluten-free toast with grilled mushrooms and tomatoes.

6. Harissa scrambled silken tofu on sourdough or gluten-free toast.

7. A green smoothie – avocado, cucumber, blueberries, water, spinach, plus a squeeze of lemon. Always opt for more vegetables than fruit. Optional extras: nuts, chia and linseeds/flaxseeds, ginger, coconut water, almond milk, cinnamon, mint, pea protein, spirulina, maca and acai powder.

simple lunches

* Leftovers! Cook more in the evening and save some for lunches, when you can add a handful of leaves.
* Batch-cooked soups.
* Buddha bowls – selections of pulses, hummus, sauerkraut, falafel, avocado, leaves, tomatoes, leftover chicken, smoked mackerel or tofu.

low-bandwidth dinners

1. Traybakes: the ultimate one-pot, low-bandwidth dinner.
2. Asian soups: ramen, a miso broth with noodles, veg and choices of meat, prawns, tofu, from Japan or *tom yum gai*, a wonderfully hot and spicy Thai soup – quick-to-make soups are especially tasty if you have some fresh chicken or vegetable stock as a base.
3. Curries: cod-and-spinach curry, cashew-and-tofu curry, Thai green curry with prawns.
4. Vegan: black bean and sweet potato chilli, roasted harissa cauliflower, miso roasted veg.
5. Stir-fries: stacks of vegetables with a protein such as chicken, prawns, tofu, egg, lean beef or beans/pulses with rice or sweet-potato noodles.
6. Dust off your slow-cooker! For low effort veggie or meat stews.

There is a free app called Whisk (whisk.com) where you can access all the recipes that I have gleaned from chefs online over the years. And I have two communities that you can access: 'Healthy and Low-Effort Midweek Meals' and 'Natural Menopause Recipes' – just search for Karen Newby or access the link via my homepage: karennewby.com. You can then create your menu plans and shopping list and link it to your preferred supermarket shop, too.

PART THREE

Symptom troubleshooting

"

THE CHANGES, THE HIGHS AND LOWS, AND THE HORMONAL SHIFTS, THERE IS POWER IN THAT...

MICHELLE OBAMA

"

INTRODUCTION

This part of the book represents my nutritional toolkit to help support the manifold symptoms of perimenopause and beyond. These are listed alphabetically, for ease of reference, and the tools include therapeutic foods, supplements and simple shifts that can help.

Cautionary supplement advice
If you are taking HRT or birth-control medication, or are on any other medication or under medical supervision, consult your healthcare practitioner before taking any food supplement. Please note that the supplement section is merely a selection of suggestions that might help a particular symptom – not all of them are to be taken at once. Do get in touch with a nutritional therapist registered with the British Association for Nutritional and Lifestyle Medicine (BANT) for a tailored protocol, taking into account your unique health needs: bant.org.uk.

aches and pains

DESCRIPTION / SYMPTOMS
Why do I feel 100, even though I'm only fifty? The problem: oestrogen again. Where there is pain, there is inflammation. There is much research on perimenopause being an inflammatory stage of life because oestrogen has a specific anti-inflammatory role in the body.[63] Reducing oestrogen levels can increase pro-inflammatory markers.

WHY IS THIS HAPPENING TO ME?
So what causes it? Aside from declining oestrogen levels, injury and processed foods, foods with a higher amount of the pro-inflammatory compound arachidonic acid – found in meat and dairy products – alcohol, caffeine, gluten, smoking, sun damage and pollution can all increase inflammation, too.

AREAS TO CONSIDER
Where there is pain, there is cortisol, because cortisol is nature's anti-inflammatory. It's also our stress hormone, which is why chronic inflammation can affect our sleep. This might be a factor to consider if you're suffering from sleep issues.

Gluten is often not very helpful either, especially if you suffer from an autoimmune condition. Published research into non-coeliac gluten sensitivity has shown it be pro-inflammatory.[64]

THERAPEUTIC FOODS
★ Increase omega-3 foods: oily fish such as salmon, sardines, trout and mackerel, linseeds, walnuts, linseed oil (not to be heated, though).
★ Omega-6 – from evening primrose oil, sesame and pumpkin seeds.
★ Vitamin C, which we don't store in the body, is essential for energy, but is also a potent antioxidant (see page 96).
★ Keep blood-sugar levels stable (see pages 48–53).
★ Turmeric and ginger are widely known for their anti-inflammatory actions (although they are heating, so be wary if you suffer from hot flushes).
★ Phytoestrogens – soya (tofu, tempeh, miso, natto, edamame beans), chickpeas, lentils, peas, ground linseed, sesame seeds,

cashews, kale, broccoli, Brussels sprouts, carrots, cabbage, cauliflower, peppers, cherries, garlic, apples, apricots, soybean sprouts, alfalfa, split peas, pinto beans and red clover tea.

✱ Include quercetin-rich foods, such as onions, apples and kale.

✱ Up foods known to help relieve and soothe pain, such as ginger, lemon balm, anise, nettle, fennel and garlic.

✱ Antioxidant-rich fruit and veg – pomegranate, blueberries, plums, red onions, beetroot, carrots, squash.

SMALL SHIFTS

· Have some days without meat and dairy products.

· Avoid cooking with vegetable oils.

· Start making pesto – oleic acid from olive oil is very healing (olive trees are some of the oldest living trees on the planet) and, when mixed with parsley, coriander, mint or basil, helps the phytonutrients from these herbs to be absorbed better.

· Start smoothie making to up your antioxidants, including vitamin C, to support the immune system.

LIFESTYLE HACKS

✱ There is anecdotal evidence of alkaloids from the nightshade family of plants worsening inflammation, especially with arthritis. This is due to the alkaloid solanine, which may aggravate arthritic pain and inflammation. These include tomatoes, aubergine, peppers, chillies and green potatoes.

✱ Start getting a fruit-and-veg box delivered to help you to eat more vegetables – it's good for juicing leftovers, too.

SUPPLEMENTS TO CONSIDER

Life & Soul Mini Capsules, Bare Biology · Turmeric Plus, Cytoplan · CT Plex, Bionutri · Evening Primrose Oil, BioCare · Acai and Chlorella, Naturya (to be added to your smoothie).

allergies and intolerances

DESCRIPTION
/ SYMPTOMS For some of my clients it can manifest as an intolerance to alcohol – sneezing after drinking – or for others, it's the onset of hayfever or eczema, asthma or intolerance to foods such as gluten.

WHY IS THIS HAPPENING TO ME? Food intolerance can start to manifest as we age, due to a reduction in digestive function (see page 58), so digestive support is needed. Oestrogen is involved with histamine production – there are oestrogen receptor sites on mast cells that release histamine; and oestrogen can also down-regulate an enzyme called DAO, which clears histamine out of the body.[65] In research on asthma, which is more prevalent in women than in men, it has been shown that oestrogen and xenoestrogens in our diet and environment, actually skews us towards more allergy.[66] So if we have oestrogen hyperstimulation or high xenoestrogens in our diet or poor oestrogen clearance from the body, this could skew towards more histamine. Histamine can also be increased by certain foods that are high in histamine or stimulate the release of histamine after eating – see lists below.

AREAS TO CONSIDER Optimizing your liver and gut health to make sure excess oestrogen is cleared from the body. Address any digestive issues including gut function. Consider high histamine foods. Start cycle tracking: do these symptoms worsen at certain times of your cycle?

THERAPEUTIC FOODS
* More phytoestrogens to help support fluctuating oestrogen levels (see list on page 91).
* Increase more of nature's antihistamine – quercetin. Found in onions, peppers, shallots, cherries, grapes and apples.
* More B6, magnesium and zinc-rich foods to support progesterone.
* Limit high-histamine foods: alcohol (especially beer and wine), anchovies, aubergine, avocados, cheese (especially aged or

fermented cheese), cider, dried fruits, fermented foods, figs, mackerel, MSG, mushrooms, processed meats, sardines, smoked fish, sour cream, yogurt, coffee, yeast, spinach, tomatoes, vinegar.
★ Also limit histamine-releasing foods: alcohol, bananas, citrus fruits, chocolate, eggs, fish, milk, papayas, pineapple, raspberries, plums, shellfish, strawberries and tomatoes.

SMALL SHIFTS
· Identify high-histamine foods and drinks that you have regularly in your diet and aim to reduce them or swap them out for alternatives.
· Remove beer (especially IPAs) and wine and swap for other drinks.
· Aim to increase your variety of foods.

LIFESTYLE HACKS
★ Opt for organic veg and fruit – this will reduce your intake of pesticides and herbicides.
★ Start tracking your symptoms. Intolerances are harder to spot than allergies as they can take up to 72 hours to manifest but a food diary can be helpful. Symptoms can include: bloating, gas, churning and urgency to go to the loo.
★ Allergies are more immediate with symptoms such as sniffles, itchy throat, gut pain and wheezing and can be life threatening in the case of anaphylaxis.

SUPPLEMENTS TO CONSIDER
Quercetin, BioCare · Rosehip Q10 with quercetin, Bionutri · Max Strength Immune Formula, Unbeelievable Health (for hay fever) · Cyto-zyme, Cytoplan · Digestive Enzymes, Wild Nutrition · S. Boulardii, Cytoplan

anxiety, panic attacks and heart palpitations

DESCRIPTION / SYMPTOMS

This really blindsides many of my clients who suddenly experience panic attacks for the first time. I've had clients call emergency services thinking they're having a heart attack with little to no explanation as to why this has happened. Well, these might be hormone related at perimenopause.

WHY IS THIS HAPPENING TO ME?

Dips in oestrogen can cause heart palpitations. When oestrogen is high, it helps to dilate our blood vessels; and when it dips, it constricts them, hence the heart palpitations and why women have a higher risk of developing high blood pressure postmenopause.[67] Progesterone is intimately connected to GABA, our calming neurotransmitter, and is indicated as one of the reasons for menopause anxiety.[68]

AREAS TO CONSIDER

Address blood-sugar control – dips in blood sugar are likely to exacerbate anxiety. This includes alcohol. I see a lot of women in my practice who, when they avoid alcohol, see a noticeable change in instances of anxiety. Zinc also is very much indicated in helping to alleviate anxiety. It's a mineral co-factor that helps to detoxify alcohol, so the more alcohol you drink, the more zinc you use up. Caffeine, too, is not helpful if you suffer from anxiety – it stimulates your heart muscle by putting your body into fight-or-flight mode. Magnesium can also help with anxiety as well as heart palpitations. It is known as nature's tranquillizer – it supports our smooth muscles, which we have no control over, like our entire cardiovascular system. As with depression, our gut has a role to play in anxiety and can help modulate incidences.[69]

* Progesterone needs vitamins B6, magnesium and zinc. B6: broccoli, Brussels sprouts, cabbage, cauliflower, kale, nuts, pumpkin, spinach, wholegrains.

* Magnesium: black beans, avocado, pumpkin, sunflower and sesame seeds, green leafy vegetables, almonds, spinach, Swiss chard; and use Epsom bath salts.

* Zinc-rich foods: oysters, prawns, lean beef, pumpkin and sesame seeds, tahini, chickpeas, brown rice, green peas, dark chocolate.

* L-theanine is an amino acid found in matcha and green tea (opt for the decaf version), which has traditionally been used to enhance relaxation.

* GABA-promoting foods: prawns, halibut, almonds, l-theanine in green tea (decaf), walnuts, soya.

* Taurine is an amino acid that helps the production of GABA: scallops, freshwater fish, turkey, chicken, seaweed, beef

* Phytoestrogens: see page 91.

* Remove tyramine-rich foods, which can stimulate adrenaline, from your evening meal; avoid bacon, cheese, chocolate, cured meats, sausages, fermented foods, yeast and wine near bedtime.

* Omega-3 for healthy blood vessels: oily fish such as salmon, sardines, trout and mackerel, linseed, walnuts.

SMALL SHIFTS

• Ditch the caffeine in favour of herbal tea, matcha and decaf green tea.

• Avoid alcohol.

• Opt for more calming swimming or yoga over HIIT.

• Eat warming, protein-rich foods to take the energy out of the head and into the digestive system e.g. ramens, tagines, curries.

LIFESTYLE
HACKS

Lisa Cory, hypnotherapist and NLP practitioner, recommends this mindfulness technique if you feel anxiety taking hold:

* Name 5 things you can see

* 4 things you can hear

* 3 things you can touch
* 2 things you can smell
* 1 thing you can taste

SUPPLEMENTS
TO CONSIDER Food-grown Magnesium, Wild Nutrition • Neuralactin Plus,
Bionutri • Epsom salts with added valerian, Westlab • MPowder
Peri-Boost • Everyday Plus, Renew Life • Cardiomega Plus,
Bionutri • Zinc Plus, Wild Nutrition

ALTERNATE NOSTRIL BREATHING, *NADI SHODHANA*

I used to do this a lot when I was practising Ashtanga yoga.
It's great to do after a yoga practice as the body is already
quietened after the *asanas* (yoga postures):

1. Sit in a comfortable position, shoulders relaxed.
2. Bring your right hand up to your face and place the forefinger
   and middle finger gently to your 'third eye' between your
   eyebrows, to act as an anchor. You will be using the thumb and
   ring finger.
3. Exhale completely, then place your right thumb over your right
   nostril.
4. Inhale through your left nostril for a count of six, then close the
   left nostril with your ring finger.
5. Pause briefly at the end of the inhale.
6. Open the right nostril and exhale through this side for a count
   of eight.
7. Inhale through the right nostril for a count of six, then close this
   nostril with your thumb again.
8. Open the left nostril and exhale through this side for a count of eight.
9. This is one round. Start off with ten rounds and then progress to
   five minutes.
10. Always finish by exhaling through the left nostril for balance.

brain fog

DESCRIPTION
/ SYMPTOMS
Why can't I remember what I came in here for? So many of us suffer from forgetfulness and an inability to process information at perimenopause and beyond. Often clients have an extremely foggy head all day and then suddenly get clarity of thought at the day's end and start doing all their admin.

**WHY IS THIS
HAPPENING
TO ME?**
Many of my clients worry that they are getting Alzheimer's, especially if they have a parent who has the condition. Alzheimer's is more common in women than in men, which is why research points to oestrogen being involved; however, Alzheimer's is also called 'diabetes of the brain' because sugar has a big role to play (research shows that if you have diabetes you have a 56 per cent greater chance of developing Alzheimer's[70]). This brain fog is likely due to dips in oestrogen – because oestrogen is neuroprotective.[71] Oestrogen also helps to modulate neural pathways that are involved with cognitive tasks. Imbalances have far-reaching effects on our cognitive function. This is where phytoestrogens can help, which have been shown in studies to improve memory.[72] Findings from the longitudinal SWAN study state that this menopause blip doesn't affect our ability for lifelong learning and that cognitive ageing might indeed be malleable.[73] So all is not lost! I must also add that stress, gut dysbiosis, dehydration and poor diet all have their role to play.

**AREAS TO
CONSIDER**
Other factors that can exacerbate the situation include sluggish circulation. The brain cells account for 25 per cent of the body's total oxygen consumption! The brain also dislikes toxins or sugar imbalances. Foggy head can be exacerbated by out-of-balance gut bacteria, especially if you suffer from recurrent thrush (see page 66). Sleep is the main time in our twenty-four-hour clock when the brain gets a good detox (see page 80).

* Our brains are made up of 60 per cent fat, so eat oily fish at least two or three times a week. Opt for small fish such as mackerel, trout or salmon to minimize mercury. Plus nuts, seeds and linseed/flaxseed oil.

* Increase phytoestrogens to help balance oestrogenic neural pathways: soya (tofu, tempeh, miso, natto, edamame beans), chickpeas, lentils, peas, ground linseed/flaxseed, sesame seeds, cashews, kale, broccoli, Brussels sprouts, carrots, cabbage, cauliflower, peppers, cherries, garlic, apples, apricots, soybean sprouts, alfalfa, split peas, pinto beans and red clover.

* Phosphatidylcholine is good for the memory neurotransmitter acetylcholine, and phosphatidylserine helps brain-cell communication. Both are found in egg yolk, tofu, oily fish, beef, sardines and fatty cheese.

* Phenylalanine converts to tyrosine for alertness, attention and focus: eat pumpkin seeds, Parmesan, soya beans, lean beef, chicken, salmon, mackerel, cod, eggs, pinto beans.

* B vitamins...or memory vitamins: found in eggs, cereals, brown rice, fish, chicken, asparagus and dark green vegetables.

* Amino acids, especially tryptophan and glutamine, which is the precursor of GABA, a calming neurotransmitter: all these are found in lean meat, poultry, nuts, seeds and avocado.

* L-theanine is an amino acid found in green tea (opt for decaf) that is traditionally used to enhance relaxation and improve concentration.

* Vitamin C is a needed for good circulation and is a powerful antioxidant that helps fight off the free radicals that can damage brain cells. Plus vitamin C supports brain health as we age: get it in citrus fruits, parsley, greens.

* Antioxidants such as flavonoids to protect the brain: from artichoke, basil, berries, celery, citrus fruits, parsley and turmeric.

* Feed your second brain – the gut. Aim for thirty-plus unique plants per week!

* Eat rosemary for remembrance (memory!).

SMALL SHIFTS

- Feed your brain with freshly made juices and smoothies.
- The brain finds it hard to deal with too much sugar.
- Be wary of how gluten affects your concentration. We are all individual, but gluten and dairy can have an opioid-like effect on the brain.

LIFESTYLE HACKS

- ✷ Keep hydrated – dehydration is linked to drops in memory and concentration.
- ✷ Exercise to help circulation and blood flow to the brain – especially inverted yoga postures.
- ✷ Try brain games: 'use it or lose it!'
- ✷ Sleep is essential to clean out the brain – see Shift 3: Rest (page 80).

SUPPLEMENTS TO CONSIDER

Life & Soul Mini Capsules, Bare Biology • Everyday Plus, Renew Life • Saccharomyces Boulardii, Allergy Research Group (if candida is suspected) • Vitamin C Complex, Bionutri • Menopause Multinutrient, BioCare • Chlorella, SunChlorella

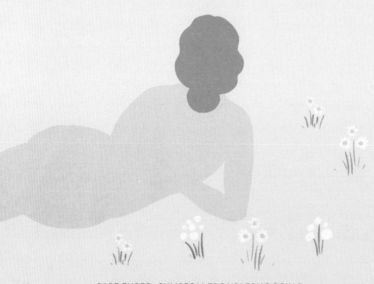

fatigue

DESCRIPTION / SYMPTOMS

Modern life has created an energy crisis – and that's before perimenopause kicks in. The reason we have this energy crisis is because the body keeps going, regardless of how much stress we are under. We've created a sophisticated biochemical and endocrine feedback system to deal with adverse events and high life-load. Although we can adapt, this is often to the detriment of our vitality.

WHY IS THIS HAPPENING TO ME?

You are a doer – and you push on through, despite your body wanting to stop. Unfortunately at perimenopause we suddenly can't source the energy that we found in our twenties and thirties. We have to reset ourselves. It's not about being lazy. It's about carving out space to actively rest. So many of us are in constant sympathetic hyper-stress mode, which is hugely energy-depleting. It's about actively moving from fight-or-flight to rest-and-digest mode.

AREAS TO CONSIDER

The key role of our thyroid is to adjust our body's energy production – our metabolic rate. In states of high stress, this organ can become dysregulated. The nervous system eats up a lot of energy, as does our brain, so a steady supply of nutrients is necessary. Inflammation and a high toxic load also use up energy. Magnesium is essential for the body's energy currency called ATP, as are B vitamins, iron and vitamin C. Remember that we don't store vitamin C in the body, so we need it daily. So often we are deficient in iron. Having tea and toast at breakfast depletes the iron from the toast, due to tannins in the tea. Coenzyme Q10 is a vitamin-like substance that is stored in the mitochondria (the energy factories in our cells), which depletes with age. Sugar is hugely energy-zapping – more rollercoasters of highs, then lows of energy.

* Vitamin-C-rich foods: leafy greens, parsley, pepper, berries, citrus fruits.
* B vitamins: eggs, cereals, brown rice, fish, asparagus and dark green vegetables.
* Magnesium-rich foods: leafy greens, pumpkin seeds, figs, black beans.
* Key thyroid-supporting foods: iodine: seaweed (kelp, nori, wakame, kombu), cod, prawns, ionized salt; selenium: Brazil nuts, sardines, halibut, prawns, beef, chicken and eggs; tyrosine: beef, pork, fish, chicken, tofu, cheese, beans, seeds, nuts; zinc: prawns, lean beef, pumpkin seeds, chickpeas; and glycine: meat, especially collagen-bone broth, fish, legumes.
* Iron-rich foods: lean beef, darker cuts of chicken, green leafy vegetables, fish, brown rice, kidney beans, chickpeas, edamame beans, quinoa, pumpkin seeds.
* Protein-rich snacks to help with afternoon energy: seeds, miso soup, falafels, smoked or beetroot hummus, guacamole, trail mix, raw chocolate.
* Alcohol affects our sleep and will exacerbate low energy the next day. It also affects the thyroid.[74]

SMALL SHIFTS

- Eat breakfast!
- A tea or coffee only lasts you till the next one. It gives you a high of energy, which then leads to a dip.
- A green smoothie at breakfast will give your body a massive micronutrient hit.
- Learn to say 'no' to personal engagements if you feel exhausted.
- Try to go to bed before you get that second wind.

* Fix yourself a fresh juice daily with your breakfast – this will give your adrenals a massive hit of all-important vitamin C, along with B vitamins, which are important for energy production, too.

* Be careful when cooking vitamin-C-rich vegetables, as this is unstable, as are B vitamins. And processed foods are not as nutrient-dense, they are more likely to lose nutrients in their processing.

* Sometimes going for a walk when we feel sleepy helps to re-energize us and refocus our intention for the day.

* Stare out of the window with a wide gaze to help to quieten and re-energize the mind.

SUPPLEMENTS
TO CONSIDER

Menopause Multinutrient, BioCare • Vitamin C Complex, Bionutri • B Complex Plus, Wild Nutrition • Liquid iron, Floradix • Iron Plus, Wild Nutrition • MPowder (any) • Maca, acai and spirulina powder, plus turmeric (to add to juice or smoothies)

Katie Light,
founder of the Light Technique, on Reiki

Everything is energy. Energy is matter, our thoughts and feelings; your spiritual / emotional well-being is the essence of who you are. We need energy to support our physical wellness, including all the functions, structures, muscles, organs and cells of our body. If our energy isn't aligned, our whole being is affected and we can get stuck in life, being unable to move forward. If we come under some form of stress, we get out of alignment and find it challenging to get back on track. Reiki energy healing involves retuning your body, mind and emotions – it's like refuelling the engine, with a full MOT and service; sparkling from the inside out, raring to go and discover the journey. This gentle yet powerful therapy works to release blocked energy held within the body and mind.

female ecology

What do I mean by 'female ecology'? I mean the areas around our vagina and vulva. Dryness, itchiness, burning, pain and frequent urinary tract infections (UTIs) are hugely distressing and uncomfortable symptoms that don't really make us want to have sex with our partners. They can put a huge strain on a relationship.

WHY IS THIS
HAPPENING
TO ME?
A healthy vaginal microbiome is quite acidic, with a pH of around of 3.6–4.5. Lowering oestrogen has an impact on the microbiota in our vagina (similar to the microbiota that we have in our gut) and the pH starts to increase. Oestrogen keeps it acidic, but, with declining levels, the pH starts to increase, making it more alkaline. This increasingly alkaline environment can make thrush and UTIs more frequent, too. Urinary-stress incontinence can also be caused by a breakdown in natural defence mechanisms.

AREAS TO
CONSIDER
For vaginal dryness, avoid substances that dry mucous membranes, such as antihistamines, alcohol, caffeine and diuretics. Phytoestrogen research has shown an increase in superficial cells of the vagina, which signify increases in circulating oestrogen.[75]

SMALL SHIFTS
- Know that this is a common issue and that a two-pronged approach working from the inside and out will help symptoms.
- Start with a high dose probiotic to help the vaginal microbiome.
- Then start increasing your vitamin C and E and omega 3 oils.
- Ensure good lubricants without parabens or perfumes, which can irritate the area.

* Phytoestrogens: (see page 91)
* Lactobaccillus probiotics to help maintain an acidic environment.
* Lubrication from:
    Omega-3 and omega-6 fats: oily fish, linseed/flaxseed oil, walnuts, sesame seeds, pumpkin seeds.
    Vitamin C: leafy green vegetables, kiwi fruit, citrus fruits.
    Vitamin E: almonds, walnuts, avocados, wheatgerm oil, sweet potato, tomatoes, salmon, mackerel, blackberries.

* Wear natural fibres.
* Talk to your partner about what is going on so they fully understand the situation. Get them to read parts of this book.
* Have regular intercourse, if it is comfortable to do so.

Bio.Me Femme V, Invivo · Bio.Me Femme C, Invivo (for thrush) · Pro-Cyan, Bio-Kult (for UTIs) · Cranberry Intensive, BioCare (for UTIs) · Lignan Plus, Bionutri · Evening Primrose Oil, BioCare · Menopause Support Formula, Nutrigold · Menophase, Higher Nature · Life & Soul Mini Capsules, Bare Biology (this also has some vitamin E as an antioxidant stabilizer for the oil) · Organic products such as YES VM vaginal moisturizer or YES WB lubricant (both available on prescription or as over the counter verisons) are pH-balanced and formulated without glycerine, glycols, parabens or perfumes.

Hair: see Skin, hair and nails (pages 144–7)
Heart palpitations: see Anxiety, panic attacks and heart palpitations (pages 113–15)

heavy periods

DESCRIPTION / SYMPTOMS

Most of us know when our periods get heavier (although what might be heavy for one woman might be normal for another) which is a common change at perimenopause; or we get prolonged periods, which according to the NHS is anything over 7 days. Usually involves flooding and/or lots of clots in periods, frequently having to change sanitary items and often suffering from low iron.

WHY IS THIS HAPPENING TO ME?

For many women, periods start to get heavier during perimenopause and last for less time. This can be due to the hyperstimulation of oestrogen, which often occurs at the start of our perimenopausal journey. Heightened oestrogen can increase the lining of the uterus meaning heavier bleeds. This also affects our progesterone – often called the period lightening hormone.[76]

AREAS TO CONSIDER

Iron deficiency is also something to consider. High blood loss is, as you would expect, associated with negative iron balance, which can lead to iron-deficiency anaemia. In a classic catch-22, iron deficiency can be a cause of a heavy flow. Do also check your intrauterine devices. Heavy flow can be a sign of hypothyroidism, which may cause a prolonged and heavy cycle. Fibroids are very sensitive to steroid hormones, in particular oestrogen, which is why they are considered an oestrogen-sensitive condition. Interestingly, they reduce in size postmenopause. If you're getting lots of clots, then fibroids could be an issue and do tend to become quite common at perimenopause; the instances in Black women are far greater than in Caucasian women.[77] One reason might be to do with vitamin D. Recent research showed that women with sufficient vitamin D status were 32 per cent less likely to suffer from fibroids. In the study only 10 per cent of Black women had sufficient vitamin D levels.[78] You can get a simple home pinprick test either via your doctor or via a private lab: www.vitamindtest.org.uk.

| THERAPEUTIC FOODS | ✱ Iron-rich foods: spinach, any other leafy greens, lean beef, darker cuts of chicken, brown rice, pulses, legumes, tofu.
| | ✱ Vitamin K: green leafy vegetables; brassicas, especially kale and broccoli; and egg yolks.
| | ✱ Increase seeds, oily fish and linseed/flaxseed oil for omega 3.
| | ✱ Support progesterone via B6, magnesium and zinc. For B6: broccoli, Brussels sprouts, cabbage, cauliflower, kale, nuts, pumpkin, spinach, wholegrains.
| | ✱ Magnesium: black beans, avocado, pumpkin, sunflower and sesame seeds, green leafy vegetables, almonds, spinach, Swiss chard.
| | ✱ Zinc: oysters, prawns, lean beef, pumpkin and sesame seeds, tahini, chickpeas, brown rice, green peas, dark chocolate.
| | ✱ Phytoestrogens (see page 91).

| LIFESTYLE HACKS | ✱ How are your stress levels? Address adrenal support to help balance cortisol (see pages 42–5).
| | ✱ If you're still regular, reduce your social engagements and harness some self care around your period.
| | ✱ Up your iron-rich food prior to your period too.

SUPPLEMENTS TO CONSIDER

Liquid iron, Floradix · Iron Plus, Wild Nutrition · Magnesium, Wild Nutrition · Menophase, Higher Nature · Menopause Support Formula, Nutrigold · Evening Primrose Oil, BioCare · Life & Soul Mini Capsules, Bare Biology · Nutrisorb Vitamin D, BioCare

SMALL SHIFTS

- Start with oestrogen balancing by supporting your liver and gut (see pages 67–71).
- Get yourself a vitamin D test if you suffer with fibroids.
- Increase phytoestrogens (see page 91).
- Up your iron-rich foods.
- Consider doing the 14-Day Cleanse (see pages 72–7).

hot flushes and night sweats

I've put hot flushes and night sweats in the same section because they are both what are known as 'vasomotor symptoms' – symptoms caused by the dilation of blood vessels in our skin to bring our body temperature down. Hot flushes are one of the most common perimenopausal symptoms – experienced by more than 70 per cent of us.[79]

WHY IS THIS
HAPPENING
TO ME?
It's all down to oestrogen – again – which also has a role to play in our body temperature control. Low oestrogen causes our temperature set point to reduce, which then stimulates adrenaline to dilate the blood vessels to stimulate flushing and sweating and bring heat down to this new 'set point' in the body. What is also important is to watch for blood-sugar lows (see pages 48–9). When we get a blood-sugar low, the body releases adrenaline to bring the blood sugar up, but at the same time it can dilate our blood vessels – hence the hot flush. I see this quite a lot with clients, whose hot flushes disappear during and after my 14-Day Cleanse (see pages 72–7) – their blood sugar has become more balanced and therefore they're dealing with fewer adrenaline surges.

AREAS TO
CONSIDER
What is your trigger? I can't tell you how useful it is to compile a hot-flush diary. When you have them, note down any of the common triggers you had that day and then a pattern should start to emerge: stimulants such as caffeine, hot drinks, alcohol, sulphites, monosodium glutamate (MSG), chocolate, sugar and spicy food. Be careful of ginger, turmeric and beetroot, because these can be warming, too. Alcohol can trigger night sweats because it's not only a stimulant, but can also cause a blood-sugar low during the night. Stress can also exacerbate flushing. If you are working at home and feel a flush coming on, stand in front of a mirror and do alternate nostril breathing (see page 115). This helps to switch the body from fight-or-flight mode to rest-and-digest mode and assists

the surges of adrenaline that can affect vasodilation (widening of the blood vessels). You can see this working in the mirror, so that when you are next at work or about to do a presentation and feel a flush coming on, you can go to a quiet space and breathe to help reduce the flush.

THERAPEUTIC FOODS

* Black cohosh has been shown in a small study of eighty women to reduce the frequency and severity of hot flushes after eight weeks of using this herb.[80] Larger studies are needed, but there does seem to be a link between a reduction in hot flushes and black cohosh.[81]
* Cooling foods: tofu, chicken, egg, apples, pears, lemon, sage tea, millet, cucumber, celery, peppermint tea, green juices.
* Phytoestrogens, especially soya, have been shown to help reduce hot flushes.[82][83] The 2015 menopause guidelines from NICE (the UK's National Institute for Health and Care Excellence) confirm that there is some evidence isoflavones may relieve vasomotor symptoms (such as flushing and temperature changes).
* Phytoestrogens: soya (tofu, tempeh, miso, natto, edamame beans), chickpeas, lentils, peas, ground linseed/flaxseed, sesame seeds, cashews, kale, broccoli, Brussels sprouts, carrots, cabbage, cauliflower, peppers, cherries, garlic, apples, apricots, soybean sprouts, alfalfa, split peas, pinto beans and red clover.

SMALL SHIFTS

- Start a hot-flush diary to see what triggers you – we are all different.
- Avoid triggers, or be mindful when you have them.
- Have a protein-rich snack before bed to help with blood-sugar lows and night-sweat adrenaline triggers.

* Research has shown vitamin E can reduce hot flushes and night sweats.[84] Food sources: evening primrose oil, almonds, sunflower seeds, avocado, spinach, chard, squash, trout.
* Vitamin C is used to help to improve collagen synthesis to keep blood vessels dilated.
* Sage is another herb that has long been used to help hot flushes. A small study of seventy-nine women showed that after four weeks flushing reduced by 50 per cent and after eight weeks by 64 per cent.[85]
* Red clover contains isoflavones, a phytoestrogen also found in soya.

LIFESTYLE HACKS

* Keep your bedroom window open to reduce the temperature in the room, so that the body has less to do to reach the new set-point temperature, should there be a dip of oestrogen in the night.
* Have lots of layers on the bed.
* Published research on acupuncture shows that it can also be a side-effect-free support for hot flushes, although research is limited to small numbers like a lot of natural medicine interventions.[86] The Menopoised magnet that can be placed on the nape of your neck, was created by acupuncturist Jo Darling and works by combining acupuncture with the power of magnets to create a natural support for hot flushes. The effectiveness of acupuncture points has been well-researched and recorded, leaving acupuncturists in no doubt which points can help with which conditions. Jo has chosen a popular heat clearing point and the Menopoised magnet simply uses a magnet as a proxy for an acupuncture needle.

SUPPLEMENTS TO CONSIDER

Black Cohosh, Higher Nature • Menopause Support, A. Vogel • Lignan Plus, Bionutri • Evening Primrose Oil, BioCare • Menophase, Higher Nature • Botanical Menopause Complex, Wild Nutrition • Female Balance, BioCare

insomnia

DESCRIPTION
/ SYMPTOMS
For many of us, sleep used to be our superpower, but as we age it starts to become more elusive. As I've already mentioned in the Rest section on page 78, the sleep stats at perimenopause are shocking, often due to dips in oestrogen and progesterone.

WHY IS THIS HAPPENING TO ME?

Night sweats, heightened anxiety, aches and pains and digestive discomfort all come into play. It's even more irritating if we're lying next to a snoring partner!

AREAS TO CONSIDER

Melatonin – known as the 'Dracula hormone' because it's released as darkness falls – is synthesized in the brain by the pineal gland, along with serotonin, which is a neurotransmitter that is also involved in sleep regulation. Melatonin is charged up during the day like a solar light and during the night it's slowly released. The body is so clever, because melatonin slows down our thinking and cools down the body, ready for restful sleep. An important raw material for both serotonin and melatonin is the protein tryptophan.

THERAPEUTIC FOODS

* Tryptophan-rich foods: chicken, turkey, salmon, kidney beans, lentils, oats, chickpeas, pumpkin seeds, sunflower seeds, tahini, walnuts, avocado, almond butter, figs, kiwis, tart cherry juice.
* Serotonin boosters: the sunshine vitamin D is needed to convert tryptophan into serotonin. Plus iron (from darker cuts of chicken, green leafy vegetables, quinoa, brown rice, lean beef, pumpkin seeds, tofu); vitamin B6 (fish, wholegrains, eggs); B12 (beef, chicken, eggs and fish, especially trout and salmon); folate (anything green and leafy, dried beans, lentils, almonds, sweet potato, beetroot, broccoli, cauliflower); and magnesium (leafy greens, pumpkin seeds, figs, black beans).

* Melatonin boosters: magnesium, zinc (lean beef, dark raw chocolate, pumpkin seeds, prawns) and folate again.

SMALL SHIFTS

- Try a light snack before bed. Foods high in the amino acid tryptophan, such as almond butter, may help you to sleep and to stop waking up in the night due to a blood-sugar low.
- Avoid alcohol too close to bedtime.
- Avoid caffeine, aside from with breakfast.
- Avoid too much tech time in the evening, and wear blue light-blocking glasses when on screen.
- Lavender and chamomile in tea improve insomnia.
- Valerian in your Epsom salts can be used as a natural sedative.

LIFESTYLE HACKS

- ★ Address cortisol levels (see pages 42–5).
- ★ Increase your phytoestrogens (see page 91)
- ★ Consider doing the 14-Day Cleanse – many clients report better sleep.
- ★ Address blood-sugar balancing (see pages 48–53).
- ★ Don't take your worries to bed. Have a worry journal by your bed or assign yourself a 'worry period' during the evening or late afternoon.
- ★ Camping is great for insomnia – away from artificial light, melatonin is released as dusk falls.

SUPPLEMENTS TO CONSIDER

Epsom Bath salts with added valerian, Westlab · Neuralactin, Bionutri · Food-grown Magnesium, Wild Nutrition · Nutrisorb Vitamin D, BioCare · Menophase, Higher Nature · Female Balance, BioCare

Irritability: see Mood swings and irritability (pages 138–40)

Dr Zoe Schaedel

from The Good Sleep Clinic

When sleep problems persist despite lifestyle changes (and optimizing hormones, where appropriate), the gold-standard treatment is Cognitive Behavioural Therapy for Insomnia, also known as CBT-I. This is a specific programme that helps to retrain your body and brain to sleep more efficiently, using a number of methods including changes to sleep scheduling, managing our minds and breaking some of the bad habits and associations that our bodies have formed. It is so much more than sleep hygiene.

CBT-I is well researched and there is lots of evidence that shows it is as effective as (or more than) any sleep medication, and the effects last for longer. It is recommended by the UK and American expert guidelines. So if you have tried tweaking your lifestyle, nutrition and hormones and your sleep is still disturbed, it may well be that CBT-I could help.

lack of libido

DESCRIPTION / SYMPTOMS

We're exhausted and anxious, and although we still look at our partners and think, 'Yes, I love you and think you're amazing, and I'd really like to have sex with you...' but the desire just isn't there. It's really distressing and can cause many problems in relationships. Refer to the section on 'female ecology' (see pages 122–3) for the *physical* symptoms related to sex, such as pain, dryness and itchiness. Here we address the *psychological* symptoms of lack of desire.

WHY IS THIS HAPPENING TO ME?

Women have many subtle dials that make us aroused, whereas men are really either OFF or ON. Not feeling good about ourselves can be a massive issue. Even brain fog (see pages 116–18) can affect our libido and lack of drive in general. Testosterone in our pre-menopause phase is the spike mid-cycle that makes us feel strong and want to have sex – in order to coincide with ovulation. Testosterone can dip at perimenopause.[87]

AREAS TO CONSIDER

Magnesium is linked to higher testosterone[88] and resistance training has been shown to increase testosterone levels in women.[89] Consider addressing weight round the middle; these central fat stores can lower testosterone by converting testosterone to more oestrogen via the enzyme aromatase (see pages 148–151).

Include omega-3 and -6 in your diet to help sex-hormone synthesis. Foods high in zinc and copper might also help – the old wives' tale of oysters being an aphrodisiac is because they contain stacks of zinc and copper. Zinc is needed for our reproductive health and copper is very much linked to arousal.

Lack of libido can be linked to tiredness – see Fatigue on page 119. Our feel-good chemical serotonin might be flagging which encourages desire – see Low mood/depression on page 134.

SMALL SHIFTS

- Exercise not only helps with flagging energy levels but will build lean muscle mass which helps support testosterone levels. Choose exercise that you enjoy – a walk with a friend or alone listening to an inspiring podcast!
- Adrenal health especially postmenopause is so important for oestrogen and testosterone production. See Shift 1, Reset on pages 40–56.

THERAPEUTIC FOODS

- ★ Phytoestrogens (see page 91).
- ★ Omega-3 foods: oily fish such as salmon, sardines, trout and mackerel, flaxseeds, walnuts, linseed oil (not to be heated, though).
- ★ Omega-6: evening primrose oil, sesame and pumpkin seeds.
- ★ Vitamin A (or via beta-carotene, which converts to vitamin A in the body): fruit and veg that is bright red, orange, yellow and green.
- ★ Vitamin C: leafy green veg, kiwi fruit, citrus fruits.
- ★ Magnesium: black beans, pumpkin, sunflower and sesame seeds, green leafy vegetables, almonds, spinach, Swiss chard.
- ★ Zinc-rich foods: oysters, prawns, lean beef, pumpkin and sesame seeds, tahini, chickpeas, brown rice, green peas, dark chocolate.
- ★ Copper-rich foods: spirulina, shiitake mushrooms, oysters, prawns, crab, leafy greens, dark chocolate.
- ★ Maca, a root originally from South America, is known for its libido-boosting benefits.[90]

LIFESTYLE HACKS

- ★ Reduce your alcohol intake to optimize your zinc status.
- ★ Get your sunshine vitamin D! Low levels have been associated with lower testosterone levels in women.[91]
- ★ Talk to your partner about how you are feeling to help them understand what's going on.

SUPPLEMENTS TO CONSIDER

Evening Primrose Oil, Nutrigold · Omega-3, Wild Nutrition · Meno Support, A. Vogel · Menopause Multinutrient, BioCare · Pea-protein powder, Pulsin · MPowder (any) · Maca, Naturya

low mood / depression

DESCRIPTION / SYMPTOMS

Many women start to have symptoms of low mood at perimenopause. We begin to lack drive and ambition and start to feel low. And it's not simply 'empty-nester syndrome', as it's sometimes shrugged off to be; it's another symptom of menopause. Recently there have been lots of news reports of women being prescribed antidepressants at menopause. However, the UK's NICE guidelines are very clear that unless you have a clinical diagnosis of depression, antidepressants should not be prescribed at menopause.[92]

WHY IS THIS HAPPENING TO ME?

Our hormones have such a big effect on our mental well-being. Oestrogen helps to support production of our 'happiness neurochemical' serotonin,[93] most of which is made in the gut,[94] so gut health is always a first port of call for me in supporting anyone with low mood or depression. Oestrogen is also linked to dopamine, which is not only related to reward, but also to motivation and pleasure, which explains feelings of lack of interest in things we used to get a lot of pleasure from. Progesterone is also called the 'everything will be okay hormone' so when we stop ovulating so frequently and progesterone is likely to be disrupted, we can start to feel low. Low mood and depression are also widely accepted in medical circles as being an inflammatory condition.[95] So helping to keep a check on inflammation will help, too. See pages 54–6.

AREAS TO CONSIDER

Our gut is our second brain (see page 66).[96] Beneficial gut bacteria also help to metabolize serotonin, our happiness neurotransmitter, and GABA, our calming neurotransmitter; and probiotics, which help to modulate mood.[97] Be in nature more. Across multiple studies, researchers have found a fascinating link between being in nature and a reduced risk of mental-health problems, along with improved mood and increased life satisfaction.[98] Research also shows a strong link between physical activity and a reduced risk of mental-health problems, including anxiety and depression.[99]

SMALL SHIFTS

- Feed your brain and your second brain as you would your body.
- Buy the best food you can afford and take time to enjoy it.
- Channel food as love. Warm, grounding food to help take energy out of the head and into the digestive system – this is an Ayurvedic remedy. Eat protein-rich broths, warm salads over raw, curries and tagines.
- Move a little – even if simply a brisk walk to and from work.

THERAPEUTIC FOODS

★ Phytoestrogens (see page 91).

★ Red clover has been shown to help with mood too.[100]

★ Gut-supporting foods: gentle plant-based fibre, fermented foods like sauerkraut and kimchi, stewed apples, ground linseed, plenty of hydration.

★ B vitamins: eggs, cereals, brown rice, fish, asparagus and dark green vegetables.

★ Zinc is involved in serotonin synthesis, and low levels have often been associated with depression.[101] Zinc-rich foods include: oysters, prawns, lean beef, pumpkin and sesame seeds, tahini, chickpeas, brown rice, green peas, dark chocolate.

★ Magnesium is associated with lower symptoms of depression:[102] eat greens, pumpkin seeds, black beans, and use Epsom salt baths.

★ Vitamin C: peppers, parsley, citrus fruits, green leafy vegetables.

★ Vitamin D is involved in serotonin synthesis,[103] which is one of the reasons why being outside is so important for mental well-being.

★ Turmeric has been shown to boost serotonin and dopamine, which both improve mood. One study found that curcumin (turmeric) improved depression symptoms.[104]

★ Smoothie-making and juicing up our antioxidants and brain-supporting vitamins and minerals.

* Quality protein-rich foods provide amino acids that are the building blocks of our brain chemicals, as well as of the immune system.
* Amino acids – especially tryptophan and glutamine, which is the precursor of GABA – are all found in lean meat, poultry, nuts, seeds, avocado.
* Omega-3 has been shown to be beneficial in cases of depression[105] – so eat salmon, trout, mackerel or sardines two or three times a week and/or vegan sources such as walnuts and linseed.

LIFESTYLE
HACKS

* Getting out into nature has a massive impact on our mental well-being[106] – I love the Japanese concept of 'forest bathing', *shinrin-yoku*.
* Walking or running seems to give us an extra boost when done in natural environments, reducing feelings of anger, fatigue and sadness. We don't even need to do it for long! Exercising in green spaces for as little as five minutes was found to improve mood and feelings of self-esteem.
* Be kind to yourself and be around people who bring you sunshine.
* 'I still want to be invited, but I'm not coming'. Learn to say no to social engagements if you don't want to go.
* Try alternate nostril breathing (see page 115). It stimulates the parasympathetic nervous system (rest and repair).

SUPPLEMENTS
TO CONSIDER

Seratonin, Allergy Research Group (not to be taken if on antidepressants) • Serotone 5-HTP, Higher Nature (not to be taken if on antidepressants) • Everyday Plus Probiotic, Renew Life • Candéa, Bio-Kult (if candida is suspected) • Saccharomyces Boulardii, Allergy Research Group (if candida is suspected) • Nutrisorb Vitamin D, BioCare • B Complex Plus, Wild Nutrition

migraines

DESCRIPTION / SYMPTOMS
Recurrent headaches lasting any time between 4 to 72 hours is more common in women than men. Migraines are typically a pounding sharp pain or throbbing, often on one side, with attacks often preceded by visual disturbances such as an aura. Migraines differ from a headache which is a more steady, dull pain starting at the base of the skull or in the forehead.

WHY IS THIS HAPPENING TO ME?
Hormone-related migraines can be linked to falling oestrogen levels, known as 'oestrogen withdrawal' especially at mid-cycle and just before menstruation when oestrogen dips.[107] At perimenopause oestrogen starts to fluctuate and dip even more (cue more migraines). Declines of oestrogen can also be linked to declines of serotonin which can also trigger migraines.

AREAS TO CONSIDER
Stress also affects our brain – it can cause our blood vessels to constrict and dilate. High-histamine foods have long been associated with migraines due to their vasodilatory affect. Tyramine can also trigger migraine (see foods to avoid below).
Support the liver, which is the primary organ for oestrogen clearance (see pages 62–3) and ensure good bowel function for serotonin support and oestrogen clearance (see pages 66–7).

THERAPEUTIC FOODS
* Phytoestrogens to help with oestrogen dips (see page 91).
* Mighty magnesium helps to reduce neuronal hyperstimulation.
* Drink plenty of liquids and slowly reduce caffeine consumption.
* Eat more anti-inflammatory foods (see pages 54–6).
* Vitamin B6 is useful for histamine breakdown and progesterone support.
* Reduce foods high in histamine and tyramine: red wine, beer, cheese, avocados, aubergine, bananas, dried fruit, fermented foods, mackerel, spinach, tomatoes, mushrooms, MSG, processed meats, vinegar, yogurt, yeast extracts.

mood swings and irritability

DESCRIPTION / SYMPTOMS — A lot of what we feel is due to a sudden overwhelming number of tasks, which normally we would be able to carry off with aplomb. Suddenly the wheels are starting to fall off, coupled with the fact that if we're not sleeping well, our irritability is going to be greater. It's not a nice feeling to be out of control, angry or tearful, often for very little reason. But there are biochemical reasons for this.

WHY IS THIS HAPPENING TO ME? — Oestrogen helps to support various hormones that have mood-boosting properties, including serotonin (our happiness brain chemical), noradrenaline (our stress hormone) and dopamine (our reward-boosting brain chemical).

When we stop having regular cycles we might not always ovulate. Ovulation is crucial for the body's main source of progesterone, which is often called our 'everything-will-be-okay hormone' – another reason why our mood might shift. And progesterone is directly linked to another calming neurochemical called GABA... so you can see how all this combines to affect our happiness levels.

AREAS TO CONSIDER — Lows of blood sugar exacerbate irritability and mood swings (see pages 48–9). As does stress or even perceived stress – suddenly we are flying off the handle because the dishwasher isn't stacked properly or shoes have been left in the hall (see pages 40–5). Stimulants (sugar, caffeine, alcohol) can make us feel even more stressed. And serotonin – our 'happiness neurotransmitter', most of which is made in the gut – requires support at this time.

THERAPEUTIC FOODS
* Protein-rich foods to help with blood-sugar balancing.
* Vitamin B6 for progesterone and serotonin synthesis: poultry, fish, wholegrains, eggs, soya beans.
* GABA-supporting foods: bananas, broccoli, almonds, fish, l-theanine in green tea (opt for decaf) and matcha.
* Phytoestrogens (see page 91).

* Adaptogens: maca, turmeric, ashwagandha, panax ginseng, Rhodiola rosea.
* More magnesium: greens, pumpkin seeds, black beans, Epsom salt baths.
* Turmeric has been shown to boost serotonin and dopamine, which both improve mood.
* Avoid refined carbs: white pasta, bread and high sugar foods.

SMALL SHIFTS

- Don't hang off your hormones – eat breakfast, drink water through the day and only have caffeine with breakfast.
- Keep your blood sugar in check by eating a protein-rich breakfast (eggs, low-sugar granola with almond or coconut yogurt and berries, smoothies with pea-protein powder and maca, scrambled tofu, avocado with roasted tomatoes and mushrooms).
- If your periods are still regular, you can pre-empt PMS mood swings by eating more protein and warming foods, as well as going easy on yourself.

LIFESTYLE HACKS

* Vagal nerve-toning: the vagal nerve is our trunk nerve and, by stimulating it, we can move from fight-or-flight to rest-and-digest mode. Try alternate nostril breathing (see page 115), which stimulates the parasympathetic nervous system (rest and repair); plus singing, gargling with a little water, and cold-water swimming.
* Choose exercise that is fun not a chore, which will help you do it more often.
* Yoga, or even just lying in Child's Pose or *Savasana*, helps to ground us to the earth.

Lisa Cory,

hypnotherapist and practitioner of NLP (neuro-linguistic programming)

A great mindfulness technique, if you feel like your head is going to explode, is as follows: STOP.

S – Stop (pause)

T – Take a breath

O – Observe your thoughts and body sensations

P – Proceed with caution

Alternatively, one of my favourite breathing exercises to help calm us down is 7/11 breathing: breathe in for 7 and out for 11.

SUPPLEMENTS TO CONSIDER Agnus Castus, Cytoplan (a herb to reduce anger when periods are regular) • Ashwagandha and Rhodiola Complex, Higher Nature or Ashwagandha Plus, Wild Nutrition (not to be used if coeliac) • B Complex Plus, Wild Nutrition • Magnesium Complex, Bionutri • Maca, Naturya • AD206, BioCare

Nails: see Skin, hair and nails (pages 144–7)
Night sweats: see Hot flushes (pages 126–8)

osteoporosis

DESCRIPTION / SYMPTOMS The word 'osteoporosis' is taken from the Greek *osteo*, meaning 'bone', and *poros*, meaning 'passage' or 'little hole'. Osteoporosis isn't a symptom of perimenopause but we are more at risk of developing it postmenopause, which is why it's important to start investing in your long-term bone health as soon as possible.

WHY IS THIS HAPPENING TO ME? Both oestrogen and progesterone work synergistically to build bone. Declining oestrogen levels trigger bone-density loss. Oestrogen, after all, is a steroid hormone that helps build things up. Phytoestrogens, due to their mimicking effect of oestrogen, have been shown to increase bone-mineral density by up to 54 per cent in menopausal women and reduce bone resorption (breakdown) by 24 per cent.[108] A recent review of randomized controlled trials on soy isoflavones again showed a beneficial effect on reducing bone-resorption markers.[109] Further analysis of fifty-two trials has shown that soy isoflavones prevent significant bone loss and increase bone-mineral density for those with normal weight across all ethnicities.[110] Bone loss can also be affected by stress – be it emotional, social, economic or illness[111] – that psychological weathering I referred to earlier (see page 14).

AREAS TO CONSIDER Calcitonin is secreted by the thyroid to keep calcium levels in the blood in check – its role is to work to reduce calcium in the blood and promote calcium absorption into the bones. The opposing parathyroid hormone leaches calcium from the bones into the blood when needed.

There is much debate about acid-forming foods that are prevalent in the Western diet, like meat, dairy products, caffeine and sugar, which cause acidosis in the body, leading to a leaching of calcium from the bones to buffer the blood.[112] I'm certainly in favour of more vegetables as calcium sources over meat and dairy to protect our bone health. But bone nutrition is about so much more than simply calcium (see other essential nutrients below). In the UK we are likely to get sufficient calcium due to the amount of dairy products that we consume. Although if we don't consume dairy, we won't become a pool on the floor without strong bones; and indeed research via the SWAN study in the US showed no link between improved bone mass and dairy intake.[113]

THERAPEUTIC FOODS

★ Phytoestrogens (see page 91).

★ I prefer to get my calcium from leafy greens, especially kale, broccoli, pak choi, watercress, tahini, tofu, tempeh, almonds, Brazil nuts and sardines (the little bones are an added source) because I am also getting the benefits of other precious bone supporting micro-minerals that are coming from these foods.

★ Vitamin D is essential to help balance calcium in the body – the best source is sunshine or supplements.

Other nutrients that are needed:

★ Phosphorus: chicken, beef, eggs, fish

★ Boron: green leafy vegetables, especially kale and spinach, chickpeas, almonds, walnuts, avocado

★ B vitamins (especially folate): eggs, cereals, brown rice, fish, chicken, asparagus and dark green vegetables

★ Vitamin K: kale, spinach, spring greens, parsley, brassicas, blueberries

★ Vitamin A (or via beta-carotene, which converts to vitamin A in the body): fruit and veg that are bright red, orange, yellow and green, and eggs and salmon

★ Vitamin C: leafy green vegetables, kiwi fruit, citrus fruits

★ Magnesium: black beans, avocado, pumpkin, sunflower and sesame seeds, green leafy vegetables, almonds, spinach, Swiss chard; plus Epsom bath salts

★ Zinc-rich foods: oysters, prawns, lean beef, pumpkin and sesame seeds, tahini, chickpeas, brown rice, green peas, dark chocolate

* Copper-rich foods: spirulina, shiitake mushrooms, oysters, prawns, crab, leafy greens, dark chocolate
* Manganese-rich foods: clams, oysters, mussels, nuts, tofu, tempeh, organic soya yogurt, leafy vegetables, black pepper

LIFESTYLE HACKS

* Optimize your digestive function to make sure that calcium and other minerals are being absorbed well.
* Start weight-bearing exercise: brisk walking, running, stair-climbing, Vinyasa yoga, resistance training with bands or weights.

SUPPLEMENTS TO CONSIDER

Osteo-B Plus, Biotics · Bone Support Formula, Nutrigold · Nutrisorb Vitamin D, BioCare · Menopause Support, A. Vogel · Lignan Plus, Bionutri · Menophase, Higher Nature

Pains: see Aches and pains (pages 109–110)
Panic attacks: see Anxiety, panic attacks and heart palpitations (pages 113–15)

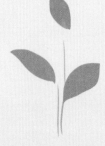

skin, hair and nails

There are benefits to having ageing eyes – I quite like looking at myself in front of the mirror without my glasses on! But joking aside, one of the main reasons for changes in skin tone is collagen loss, which can amount to 30 per cent at menopause. Oestrogen is our youth serum. In addition to the loss of collagen, low oestrogen / high testosterone can cause changes in our skin, such as facial hair and spots, too. The joys of womanhood!

WHY IS THIS HAPPENING TO ME?

Let's start with skin elasticity. Collagen is the scaffolding, if you like, for our skin and as this declines, so does our skin tone. But much can be done to help, with food and supplements.

Adult acne can arise, due to changes in our testosterone-to-oestrogen ratio. As oestrogen declines, testosterone can become more dominant, as the rate at which it is made doesn't alter so much, leading to facial hair, hair loss and acne.

Eczema in Greek literally means 'to boil over'. Eczema is linked to inflammation in the body, as are conditions such as rosacea and psoriasis.

AREAS TO CONSIDER

When it comes to spots, processed foods and sugar have a big role to play. A high-carbohydrate diet can stimulate more sebum production[114] (see the blood-sugar section on pages 48–53).

Up your zinc-rich foods. Zinc is involved in keeping testosterone in check.[115] Processed foods can lead to inflammation and spots, especially around the chin area.

For collagen synthesis, we need a steady supply of protein and vitamin C – which we don't store in the body very well.

Lack of vitamin A can cause hyperkeratinization, which blocks sebum glands and can cause dry skin.

Research on patients with acne has shown low vitamins A and E, leading to conclusions that these nutrients are involved with the pathogenesis of acne.[116]

Omega-3 is often low in our diet, but can really help with dry skin, bobbles on the backs of the arms and cracked heels. It also exerts anti-inflammatory effects, which is useful in cases of acne, eczema, rosacea and psoriasis.[117]

Antioxidant-rich diets will help with inflammation in cases of eczema, rosacea and psoriasis. Have a slice of lemon in water on waking to rehydrate your skin.

Justine Masters,

a skincare specialist, shares her top tips for midlife skin

- Always wear an SPF. 'This is Ibiza circa 1985,' she jokes with clients when discussing skin ageing.

- Use a gentle cleanser without fragrance, parabens and sulphites, which can irritate the skin.

- Don't cleanse in the shower – the water is often way too hot and we don't cleanse for long enough.

- Don't use harsh scrubs. Use enzyme powders or gentle alpha hydroxy acid (AHA) as they are gentler on the skin.

- Apply serums to slightly damp skin apart from Vitamin A – this should be applied onto dry skin.

- Ditch the wipes – they do not get all your makeup off and do not allow for a deep clean.

- Use hydration sprays to lock in moisture.

THERAPEUTIC FOODS FOR SKIN ELASTICITY

★ Top collagen foods: bone broth, egg whites, chicken, meat and fish.

★ Omega-3 for skin softness, from oily fish, nuts (especially walnuts) and their oils.

★ Vitamin C is needed for the production of collagen – so get juicing.

★ Bioflavonoids help collagen synthesis – from plums, rosehips, pomegranates.

★ Rutin stabilizes veins under the skin – from asparagus, buckwheat, cherries, grapes, oranges.

★ Hyaluronic acid in supplement form keeps the skin hydrated (dry skin exaggerates the lines).

★ Increase vitamin A – from green leafy vegetables, orange-coloured fruit and veg (mango, sweet potato, carrot, apricot, peppers), legumes, seeds, egg yolks.

★ Antioxidant vitamin E – from nuts, seeds, eggs, wheatgerm, green leafy vegetables.

★ Increase other antioxidants (such as vitamin C, phytonutrients, vitamin E and omega-3) to help quench free radicals, which play havoc with our skin.

★ Water: keep hydrated to assist with fine lines and dry skin.

THERAPEUTIC FOODS FOR MENOPAUSE ACNE

★ Limit your intake of high-fat and processed foods, such as margarine, crisps, pastries, fried foods, sweets, chocolate.

★ Reduce your dairy intake and see if this has an effect.

★ Increase zinc-rich foods: prawns and other crustaceans, lean beef, sesame and pumpkin seeds, dark raw chocolate.

★ Eat more protein and good-fat-rich foods to help balance blood-sugar levels (see blood sugar balancing on pages 48–51).

★ Support liver function (see the Cleanse section on pages 72–7).

THERAPEUTIC FOODS FOR HAIR LOSS

✱ More protein, zinc and omega-3 fats will help with hair loss and brittle nails (the whites on nails can be a sign of low zinc).

✱ Vitamin C for connective tissue, of which hair is one.

✱ Increase iron-rich foods which can help with hair loss; hair loss can also be due to anaemia or thyroid issues, so consult your doctor, too.

LIFESTYLE HACKS

✱ Have a slice of lemon in water on waking to rehydrate your skin.

✱ Get used to drinking water. Drink a small glass every half an hour of so, not too much around food.

✱ Wear an SPF – through your moisturizer or sun cream.

SUPPLEMENTS TO CONSIDER

Life & Soul Mini Capsules, Bare Biology • Evening Primrose Oil, BioCare (good for eczema and rosacea) • Collagen Complex, BioCare • Ultimate Collagen+, Ingenious Beauty • Skinful Pure Marine Collagen Powder, Bare Biology • Everyday Plus Probiotic, Renew Life • Vitamin C Complex, Bionutri • Turmeric Plus, Cytoplan

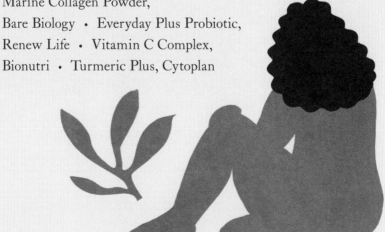

weight gain

For many of my clients, sudden weight gain is a real problem. Suddenly we lose our waist and we start to shift to what's known as a male pattern of weight gain (around the middle) due to declining oestrogen levels. Our metabolic rate slows and our insulin sensitivity declines due to lower levels of oestrogen. Plus our stress levels are often super high as we're spinning many plates, which leads to the worry waist – regardless of perimenopause! More stress leads to that frazzled feeling which means we reach for more stimulants and less helpful food to get us through the day. If this wasn't enough, research into the hunger hormone ghrelin has shown that it can be hyper-stimulated at perimenopause, meaning we're more hungry and susceptible to cravings.[118] Leptin, our 'we're no longer hungry' hormone can also be impaired according to published research, so we have no off switch!

The problem is that central weight gain at perimenopause increases inflammation and also affects our ability to control insulin. It also is a risk factor for breast cancer.[119] So getting weight-gain in check is incredibly important and will help support your midlife vitality no end. You can do my 14-Day Cleanse (see pages 72–7) as a weight-loss kick-start, but don't worry if that requires too much organization at the present time.

WHY IS THIS HAPPENING TO ME?
We have to approach weight loss differently at midlife. No amount of calorie-counting or cardio exercise will shift that weight round the middle – it's because of our hormones! These central fat cells start to interfere with our hormones and our immune system. They are not the same as other traditional fat storage cells found in the hips or butt or legs. This is why our weight-loss toolbox from our 30s and early 40s just doesn't work any more!

Fat is your friend! Especially essential fatty acids like omega-3. Fat is essential for our satiety levels and for the absorption of certain vitamins (A, E, D and K), which need fat in order to be absorbed. Blood-sugar control is also so important (see pages 48–53).

No need for calorie counting, but portion control for carbohydrates such as white rice will help – aim for a handful of dried rice per portion. *When* you consume your calories is very important: eat with the path of the sun. Breakfast is key and has a positive effect on the number of calories consumed later in the day.

* Include a source of protein in every meal to help maintain steady energy levels and reduce hunger and cravings.
* Phytoestrogens: soya (tofu, tempeh, miso, natto, edamame beans), chickpeas, lentils, peas, ground linseed/flaxseed, sesame seeds, cashews, kale, broccoli, Brussels sprouts, carrots, cabbage, cauliflower, peppers, cherries, garlic, apples, apricots, soybean sprouts, alfalfa, split peas, pinto beans and red clover.
* Enjoy breakfast.
* Start smoothie making and juicing to give your body a micronutrient hit to help with energy. Aim for more vegetables than fruit.

SMALL SHIFTS
- Don't diet! Calorie restriction is so last millennium.
- Fast overnight for twelve to fourteen hours.
- Micro-fast between meals.
- Eat with the path of the sun – eating most your food at the end of the day means it's more likely to be laid down as fat.
- Take time to eat and chew well – let your body tell you it is satisfied (usually around twenty minutes).

* Eat a rainbow of colours from fruit and vegetables daily – aim for a 2:6 ratio of fruit to veg.
* Remember that fat gain around the middle increases inflammation, which then increases cortisol (see the Worry Waist on page 52). Increasing anti-inflammatory foods will help, such as omega-3 fats,[120] linseed/flaxseed oil, nuts and seeds, as well as brightly coloured fruits and vegetables, which contain lots of antioxidants that help support our immune system.
* Eat as much junk food as you like – *if* you cook it yourself! Be wary of processed energy-dense foods that are low in nutrients.
* Avoid gluten-rich carbs, such as pasta and bread (do view pasta and rice as sugar), and opt for complex carbs, such as oats, brown rice, quinoa, pulses and brightly coloured vegetables.
* Reduce refined carbs to stop those blood-sugar rollercoasters (see pages 48–53).
* Address any emotional eating cues (see page 50).
* Reduce stimulants and stress (see pages 40–6).
* Support hormone balance (see the Cleanse section on pages 72–7).

LIFESTYLE HACKS
* Ditch the diet fizzy drinks and fake sugar – they create more cravings.
* Junk food is okay to eat occasionally, just don't put these foods on a pedestal!
* Don't frame days as good or bad – consistency over perfection.
* If you're hungry, drink a glass of water; you might be thirsty.
* If you're hungry and you don't want to eat an apple…then you're probably not hungry (see the section on emotional eating on page 50).
* Movement while fasting helps metabolic flexibility and fat burning.
* Build lean muscle mass – muscles burn more energy.

Menopause Multinutrient, BioCare • Everyday Plus Probiotic, Renew Life • Cyto-Zyme, Cytoplan (for digestive support) • Organic powdered spirulina / chlorella / maca (for additional boosts in smoothies) • Organic pea-protein powder, Pulsin (to pop into your smoothie) • Life & Soul Mini Capsules, Bare Biology • Evening Primrose Oil, BioCare

Lucy Pinto,

founder of TheBox, Brighton

Resistance training is now more important than ever at our perimenopause stage. We aren't talking 100kg [220lb] deadlifts here – resistance training can be anything from body-weight lunges, squats to weighted compound moves and, of course, the use of trusty resistance bands. A good burst of cardio is great to build into your programme, but ask yourself, 'Is this serving me and my body well?' Think LISS (Low Intensity Steady State) over HIIT (High Intensity Interval Training). You'll be protecting your bones from early-stage osteoporosis and focusing on building strength. Rest is also part of the process. We don't need to be hitting personal bests every month – movement should be fun; enjoy the process.

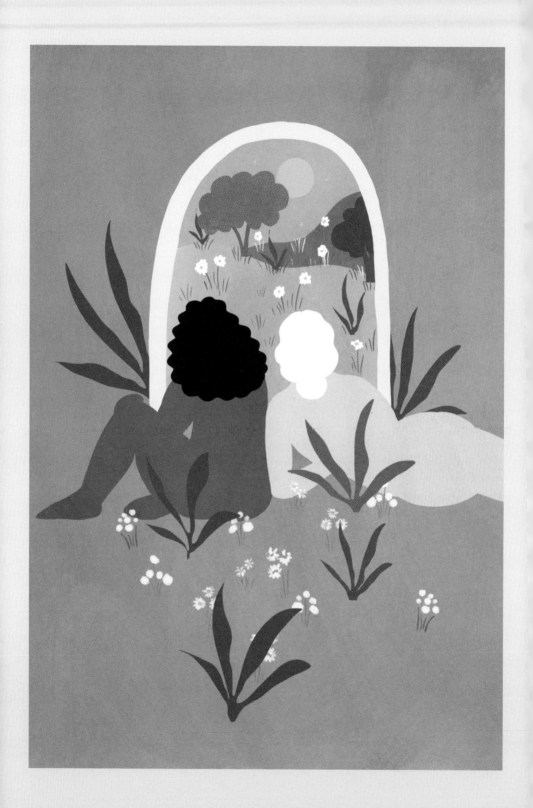

thank you

I hope this book helps you reconnect to yourself after years of looking after everyone else. I know it might be a lot of information to take in initially but it will become second nature before too long. Creating change in ourselves affects everything and everyone around us, so watch out world!

Thank you to my amazing contributors who have added their thoughts and professional advice offering up new perspectives and tools outside of nutrition to help you navigate this life stage:

Karen Arthur – Menopause Whilst Black
reddskin.co.uk/menopausewhilstblack
Lisa Cory – Hypnotherapist and NLP Practitioner
mynewperspective.co.uk
Jo Darling – Acupuncturist and Menopoised Founder
menopoised.co.uk
Dr Olivia Hum – Specialist Menopause GP, Women's Health Sussex
womenshealthsussex.com
Katie Light – The Light Technique
thelighttechnique.com
Justine Masters Skincare / justinemasters.london
Lucy Pinto – TheBox Founder and PT / theboxfit.co.uk
Jess Rad – The WomenHood / thewomenhood.com
Dr Zoe Schaedel – GP and CBT-I specialist, The Good Sleep Clinic
goodsleep.clinic

I'm so honoured that you have picked up this book (and read to the end!) and I close by wishing you abundant health and happiness through this journey called menopause.

index

references

PART 1

1 https://www.ons.gov.uk/peoplepopulationandcommunity/
birthsdeathsandmarriages/
conceptionandfertilityrates/bulletins/
childbearingforwomenbornindifferentyearsenglandand
wales/2019

2 Global Gender Gap Report, March 2021, World
Economic Forum

3 www.ipsos.com/sites/default/files/ct/news/
documents/2020-10/menopause-and-the-workplace-ipsos-
mori.pdf

4 www.ipsos.com/sites/default/files/ct/news/
documents/2020-10/ menopause-and-the-workplace-
ipsos-mori.pdf

5 https://www.npeu.ox.ac.uk/assets/downloads/mbrrace-
uk/reports/maternal-report-2021/MBRRACE-UK_
Maternal_Report_2021_-_FINAL_-_WEB_VERSION.
pdf

6 Prior, J.C., Hitchcock, C.L., 'The endocrinology of
perimenopause: need for a paradigm shift', Front Biosci
(Schol Ed), (1 Jan 2011), 3: 474–86; doi: 10.2741/s166;
PMID: 21196391

7 Wypych K, Kuźlik R, Wypych P. [Hormonal
abnormalities in women with breast cysts]. Ginekologia
Polska. 2002 Nov;73(11):1117-1125. PMID: 12722409.

8 Borahay MA, Asoglu MR, Mas A, Adam S, Kilic
GS, Al-Hendy A. Estrogen Receptors and Signaling
in Fibroids: Role in Pathobiology and Therapeutic
Implications. Reprod Sci. 2017;24(9):1235-1244.
doi:10.1177/1933719116678686

9 Mauvais-Jarvis F, Clegg DJ, Hevener AL. The role
of estrogens in control of energy balance and glucose
homeostasis. Endocr Rev. 2013 Jun;34(3):309-38. doi:
10.1210/er.2012-1055. Epub 2013 Mar 4. PMID: 23460719;
PMCID: PMC3660717

10 Prior JC. The ageing female reproductive axis II:
ovulatory changes with perimenopause. Novartis Found
Symp. 2002;242:172-86; discussion 186-92. PMID:
11855687.

11 www.ncbi.nlm.nih.gov/pmc/articles/PMC4335177/

12 www.ncbi.nlm.nih.gov/pmc/articles/PMC4171725/

13 https://www.ncbi.nlm.nih.gov/pmc/articles/
PMC8538505/

14 https://www.ncbi.nlm.nih.gov/pmc/articles/PMC2311418/

15 https://www.researchgate.net/publication/7711455_
Ovarian_Aging_and_the_Perimenopausal_
Transition_The_Paradox_of_Endogenous_Ovarian_
Hyperstimulation

16 Martinelli, P.M., Sorpreso, I.C.E., Raimundo, R.D.
et al., 'Heart rate variability helps to distinguish the
intensity of menopausal symptoms: A prospective,
observational and transversal study', PLoS One (15 Jan
2020), 15(1): e0225866; doi: 10.1371/journal. pone.0225866;
Erratum in PLoS One (6 Feb 2020), 15(2): e0229094;
PMID: 31940354; PMCID: PMC6961890

17 www.ncbi.nlm.nih.gov/pmc/articles/PMC6226272/

18 https://pubmed.ncbi.nlm.nih.gov/31001050/

19 https://www.ncbi.nlm.nih.gov/pmc/articles/
PMC3816846/

20 https://www.ncbi.nlm.nih.gov/pmc/articles/
PMC2689796/

21 https://www.ncbi.nlm.nih.gov/pmc/articles/
PMC7215544/

22 'Uterine fibroids: When is treatment with hormones
considered?' (updated 24 Mar 2020); available at: www.
ncbi.nlm.nih.gov/books/NBK279532/

23 www.ncbi.nlm.nih.gov/pmc/articles/PMC6226272/

24 https://pubmed.ncbi.nlm.nih.gov/11855687/

25 Mohanty, S.S., Mohanty, P.K., 'Obesity as potential
breast cancer risk factor for postmenopausal women',
Genes Dis (10 Sep 2019), 8(2): 117–23; doi: 10.1016/j.
gendis.2019.09.006; PMID: 33997158; PMCID:
PMC8099684

26 pubmed.ncbi.nlm.nih.gov/16034185/

27 https://www.ncbi.nlm.nih.gov/pmc/articles/PMC3197715/

28 https://www.ncbi.nlm.nih.gov/pmc/articles/
PMC8099684/

29 Ibid.

30 https://www.ncbi.nlm.nih.gov/pmc/articles/
PMC5509974/

31 https://pubmed.ncbi.nlm.nih.gov/28778332/

32 https://www.nature.com/articles/s41574-019-0273-8

PART 2

[33] https://www.ncbi.nlm.nih.gov/pmc/articles/PMC4391691/

[34] Yan, H., Yang, W., Zhou, F. et al., 'Estrogen Improves Insulin Sensitivity and Suppresses Gluconeogenesis via the Transcription Factor Foxo1', Diabetes (Feb 2019), 68(2): 291–304, doi: 10.2337/ db18-0638; Epub 28 Nov 2018; PMID: 30487265; PMCID: PMC6341301

[35] McCarthy, M., Raval, A.P., 'The peri-menopause in a woman's life: a systemic inflammatory phase that enables later neurodegenerative disease', J Neuroinflammation (2020), 17:317; doi.org/10.1186/s12974-020-01998-9

[36] Simopoulos, A.P., 'An Increase in the Omega-6/Omega-3 Fatty Acid Ratio Increases the Risk for Obesity, Nutrients (2 Mar 2016), 8(3): 128; doi: 10.3390/nu8030128; PMID: 26950145; PMCID: PMC4808858

[37] Lerner, A., Shoenfeld, Y., Matthias, T., 'Adverse effects of gluten ingestion and advantages of gluten withdrawal in nonceliac autoimmune disease', Nutr Rev (1 Dec 2017), 75(12): 1046–58; doi: 10.1093/nutrit/nux 054; PMID: 29202198

[38] Flanagan, A., Bechtold, D.A., Pot, G.K., Johnston, J.D., 'Chrono-nutrition: From molecular and neuronal mechanisms to human epidemiology and timed feeding patterns', J Neurochem (Apr 2021), 157(1): 53–72; doi: 10.1111/jnc.15246; Epub 10 Dec 2020; PMID: 33222161

[39] Paoli, A., Tinsley, G., Bianco, A., Moro, T., 'The Influence of Meal Frequency and Timing on Health in Humans: The Role of Fasting', Nutrients (28 Mar 2019), 11(4): 719, doi: 10.3390/ nu11040719, PMID: 30925707; PMCID: PMC 6520689

[40] Cresci GA, Bawden E. Gut Microbiome: What We Do and Don't Know. Nutr Clin Pract. 2015;30(6):734-746. doi:10.1177/0884533615609899

[41] Foster, J.A., McVey Neufeld, K.A., 'Gut-brain axis: how the microbiome influences anxiety and depression', Trends Neurosci (May 2013), 36(5): 305–12; doi: 10.1016/j.tins.2013.01.005; Epub 4 Feb 2013; PMID: 23384445

[42] Fasano, A., 'Zonulin, regulation of tight junctions, and autoimmune diseases', Ann N Y Acad Sci (Jul 2012), 1258(1): 25–33; doi: 10.1111/j.1749-6632.2012.06538.x; PMID: 22731712; PMCID: PMC3384703

[43] Biesiekierski, J.R., Iven, J., 'Non-coeliac gluten sensitivity: piecing the puzzle together', United European Gastroenterol J (Apr 2015), 3(2): 160–5; doi: 10.1177/2050640615578388; PMID: 25922675; PMCID: PMC4406911

[44] https://www.ncbi.nlm.nih.gov/pmc/articles/PMC4335177/

[45] Ibid.

[46] National Health Interview Survey, 2015 https://www.cdc.gov/nchs/products/databriefs/db286.htm

[47] Aoyama, S., Shibata, S., 'Time-of-Day-Dependent Physiological Responses to Meal and Exercise', Front Nutr (28 Feb 2020), 7: 18; doi: 10.3389/fnut.2020.00018; PMID: 32181258; PMCID: PMC7059348

[48] Seelig E, Keller U, Klarhöfer M, et al. Neuroendocrine regulation and metabolism of glucose and lipids in primary chronic insomnia: a prospective case-control study. PLoS One. 2013;8(4):e61780. Published 2013 Apr 12. doi:10.1371/journal.pone.0061780

[49] Bernatoniene, J., Kazlauskaite, J.A., Kopustinskiene, D.M., 'Pleiotropic Effects of Isoflavones in Inflammation and Chronic Degenerative Diseases', Int J Mol Sci (26 May 2021), 22(11): 5656; doi: 10.3390/ijms22115656; PMID: 34073381; PMCID: PMC8197878

[50] Petrine, J.C.P., Del Bianco-Borges, B., 'The influence of phytoestrogens on different physiological and pathological processes: An overview', Phytother Res (Jan 2021), 35(1): 180–97; doi: 10.1002/ptr.6816; Epub 11 Aug 2020; PMID: 32780464

[51] da Silva Schmitz, I., Schaffer, L.F., Busanello, A. et al., 'Isoflavones prevent oxidative stress and inhibit the activity of the enzyme monoamine oxidase in vitro', Mol Biol Rep (Apr 2019), 46(2): 2285–92; doi: 10.1007/s11033-019-04684-z; Epub 12 Feb 2019; PMID: 30756334

[52] Sathyapalan, T., Aye, M., Rigby, A.S. et al., 'Soy isoflavones improve cardiovascular disease risk markers in women during the early menopause', Nutr Metab Cardiovasc Dis (Jul 2018), 28(7):691–7; doi: 10.1016/j.numecd.2018.03.007; Epub 10 Apr 2018; PMID: 29739677

[53] Chen, L.R., Ko, N.Y., Chen, K.H., 'Isoflavone Supplements for Menopausal Women: A Systematic Review', Nutrients (4 Nov 2019), 11(11): 2649; doi: 10.3390/nu11112649; PMID: 31689947; PMCID: PMC6893524

[54] Douglas, C.C., Johnson, S.A., Arjmandi, B.H., 'Soy and its isoflavones: the truth behind the science in breast cancer', Anticancer Agents Med Chem (Oct 2013), 13(8): 1178–87; doi: 10.2174/18715206113139990320; PMID: 23919747

[55] Qiu, S., Jiang, C., 'Soy and isoflavones consumption and breast cancer survival and recurrence: a systematic review and meta-analysis', Eur J Nutr (Dec 2019), 58(8): 3079–90; doi: 10.1007/ s00394-018-1853-4; Epub 31 Oct 2018; PMID: 30382332

[56] Wei, Y., Lv, J., Guo, Y. et al, China Kadoorie Biobank Collaborative Group, 'Soy intake and breast cancer risk: a prospective study of 300,000 Chinese women and a dose-response meta-analysis', Eur J Epidemiol (Jun 2020),

35(6): 567–78; doi: 10.1007/s10654-019-00585-4; Epub 21 Nov 2019; PMID: 31754945; PMCID: PMC7320952

[57] Reddy, N.R., Pierson, M.D., 'Reduction in antinutritional and toxic components in plant foods by fermentation', Food Research International (1994), 27(3): 281–90; ISSN 0963-9969; doi. org/10.1016/0963-9969(94)90096-5

[58] Paucar-Menachoa, L.M., Berhowc, M.A., Gontijo Mandarinod, J.M. et al., 'Optimisation of germination time and temperature on the concentration of bioactive compounds in Brazilian soybean cultivar BRS 133 using response surface methodology', Food Chemistry (2010), 119: 636–42

[59] EFSA, 'Risk assessment for peri-and post-menopausal women taking food supplements containing isolated isoflavones', EFSA journal (2015)

[60] Otun, J., Sahebkar, A., Östlundh, L. et al., 'Systematic Review and Meta-analysis on the Effect of Soy on Thyroid Function', Sci Rep (2019), 9:3964; doi. org/10.1038/s41598-019-40647-x

[61] https://www.ncbi.nlm.nih.gov/pmc/articles/PMC4354933/

[62] Petroski, W., Minich, D.M., 'Is There Such a Thing as "Anti- Nutrients"? A Narrative Review of Perceived Problematic Plant Compounds', Nutrients (24 Sept 2020), 12(10): 2929; doi: 10.3390/ nu12102929; PMID: 32987890; PMCID: PMC7600777

PART 3

[63] McCarthy, M., Raval, A.P., 'The peri-menopause in a woman's life: a systemic inflammatory phase that enables later neurodegenerative disease', J Neuroinflammation (2020), 17: 317; doi.org/10.1186/s12974-020-01998-9

[64] Lerner, A., Shoenfeld, Y., Matthias, T., 'Adverse effects of gluten ingestion and advantages of gluten withdrawal in nonceliac autoimmune disease', Nutr Rev (1 Dec 2017), 75(12): 1046–58; doi: 10.1093/nutrit/nux 054; PMID: 29202198

[65] Narita, S., Goldblum, R.M., Watson, C.S. et al., 'Environmental estrogens induce mast cell degranulation and enhance IgE-mediated release of allergic mediators', Environ Health Perspect (Jan 2007), 115(1): 48–52; doi: 10.1289/ehp.9378; PMID: 17366818; PMCID: PMC 1797832

[66] www.ncbi.nlm.nih.gov/pmc/articles/PMC3537328/

[67] Reslan, O.M., Khalil, R.A., 'Vascular effects of estrogenic menopausal hormone therapy', Rev Recent Clin Trials (Feb 2012), 7(1): 47–70; doi: 10.2174/157488712799363253; PMID: 21864249; PMCID: PMC3227781

[68] Sovijit, W.N., Sovijit, W.E., Pu, S. et al., 'Ovarian progesterone suppresses depression and anxiety-like behaviors by increasing the Lactobacillus population of gut microbiota in ovariectomized mice', Neurosci Res (22 Apr 2019), S0160-0102(19)30142-7; doi: 10.1016/j.neures.2019.04.005; Epub: ahead of print; PMID: 31022413

[69] Huang, F., Wu, X., 'Brain Neurotransmitter Modulation by Gut Microbiota in Anxiety and Depression', Front Cell Dev Biol (11 Mar 2021), 9: 649103; doi: 10.3389/fcell.2021.649103; PMID: 33777957; PMCID: PMC7991717

[70] Cholerton, B., Baker, L.D., Montine, T.J., Craft, S,. 'Type 2 Diabetes, Cognition, and Dementia in Older Adults: Toward a Precision Health Approach', Diabetes Spectr (Nov 2016), 29(4): 210–19; doi: 10.2337/ds16-0041; PMID: 27899872; PMCID: PMC5111529

[71] Arevalo, M.A., Azcoitia, I., Garcia-Segura, L.M., 'The neuroprotective actions of oestradiol and oestrogen receptors', Nat Rev Neurosci (Jan 2015), 16(1): 17–29; doi: 10.1038/nrn3856; Epub 26 Nov 2014; PMID: 25423896

[72] Sumien, N., Chaudhari, K., Sidhu, A., Forster, M.J., 'Does phytoestrogen supplementation affect cognition differentially in males and females?', Brain Res (13 Jun 2013), 1511. 123–7, doi. 10.1016/j.brainres.2013.02.013; Epub 13 Feb 2013; PMID: 23415935; PMCID: PMC3677816

[73] Karlamangla, A.S., Lachman, M.E., Han, W. et al., 'Evidence for Cognitive Aging in Midlife Women: Study of Women's Health Across the Nation', PLoS One (3 Jan 2017), 12(1): e0169008; doi: 10.1371/journal.pone.0169008; PMID: 28045986; PMCID: PMC5207430

[74] Balhara, Y.P., Deb, K.S., 'Impact of alcohol use on thyroid function', Indian J Endocrinol Metab (July 2013), 17(4): 580–7; doi: 10.4103/2230-8210.113724; PMID: 23961472; PMCID: PMC3743356

[75] Chiechi, L.M., Putignano, G., Guerra, V. et al., 'The effect of a soy rich diet on the vaginal epithelium in postmenopause: A randomized double blind trial', Maturitas (2003), 45: 241–6; 10.1016/S0378-5122(03)00080-X

[76] https://www.ncbi.nlm.nih.gov/books/NBK279293/

[77] McWilliams, M.M., Chennathukuzhi, V.M., 'Recent Advances in Uterine Fibroid Etiology', Semin Reprod Med (Mar 2017), 35(2): 181–9; doi: 10.1055/s-0037-1599090; Epub 9 Mar 2017; PMID: 28278535; PMCID: PMC5490981

[78] Baird, D.D., Hill, M.C., Schectman, J.M., Hollis, B.W., 'Vitamin d and the risk of uterine fibroids', Epidemiology (May 2013), 24(3): 447–53; doi: 10.1097/EDE.0b013e31828acca0; PMID: 23493030; PMCID: PMC 5330388

[79] Bansal, R., Aggarwal, N., 'Menopausal Hot Flashes: A Concise Review', J Midlife Health (Jan–Mar 2019), 10(1): 6–13; doi: 10.4103/ jmh.JMH_7_19; PMID: 31001050; PMCID: PMC 6459071

[80] Mehrpooya, M., Rabiee, S., Larki-Harchegani, A. et al., 'A comparative study on the effect of "black cohosh" and "evening primrose oil" on menopausal hot flashes', J Educ Health Promot (2018), 7: 36; doi: 10.4103/jehp.jehp_81_17

[81] Shahnazi, M., Nahaee, J., Mohammad-Alizadeh-Charandabi, S., Bayatipayan, S., 'Effect of black cohosh (cimicifuga racemosa) on vasomotor symptoms in postmenopausal women: a randomized clinical trial', J Caring Sci (1 Jun 2013), 2(2): 105–13, doi: 10.5681/jcs.2013.013, PMID: 25276716; PMCID: PMC4161092

[82] Chen, M.N., Lin, C.C., Liu, C.F., 'Efficacy of phytoestrogens for menopausal symptoms: a meta-analysis and systematic review', Climacteric (Apr 2015), 18(2): 260–9; doi: 10.3109/13697137.2014.966241; Epub 1 Dec 2014; PMID: 25263312; PMCID: PMC4389700

[83] Taku, K., Melby, M.K., Kronenberg, F. et al., 'Extracted or synthesized soybean isoflavones reduce menopausal hot flash frequency and severity: systematic review and meta-analysis of randomized controlled trials', Menopause (2012)19(7):776–90

[84] Ziaei, S., Kazeminejad, A., Zareai, M., 'The Effect of Vitamin E on Hot Flashes in Menopausal Women', Gynecol Obstet Invest (2007), 64: 204–7; doi: 10.1159/000106491

[85] Bommer, S., Klein, P., Suter, A., 'First time proof of sage's tolerability and efficacy in menopausal women with hot flushes', Adv Ther (Jun 2011), 28(6):490–500; doi: 10.1007/s12325-011- 0027-z; Epub 16 May 2011; PMID: 21630133

[86] Lund KS, Siersma V, Brodersen J, Waldorff FB. Efficacy of a standardised acupuncture approach for women with bothersome menopausal symptoms: a pragmatic randomised study in primary care (the ACOM study). BMJ Open. 2019 Feb 19;9(1): e023637. doi: 10.1136/bmjopen-2018-023637. PMID: 30782712; PMCID: PMC6501989.

[87] pubmed.ncbi.nlm.nih.gov/7714119/

[88] www.ncbi.nlm.nih.gov/pmc/articles/PMC3958794/

[89] pubmed.ncbi.nlm.nih.gov/9660159/

[90] Brooks, N.A., Wilcox, G., Walker, K.Z. et al., 'Beneficial effects of Lepidium meyenii (Maca) on psychological

symptoms and measures of sexual dysfunction in postmenopausal women are not related to estrogen or androgen content', Menopause (Nov–Dec 2008),15(6): 1157–62; doi: 10.1097/gme.0b013e3181732953; PMID: 18784609

[91] www.ncbi.nlm.nih.gov/pmc/articles/PMC5218632/

[92] www.nice.org.uk/guidance/ng23/ifp/chapter/managing-your-symptoms#low-mood

[93] Hudon Thibeault, A.A., Sanderson, J.T., Vaillancourt, C., 'Serotonin-estrogen interactions: What can we learn from pregnancy?', Biochimie (Jun 2019), 161: 88–108; ISSN 0300-9084; doi.org/10.1016/j.biochi.2019.03.023

[94] Banskota, S., Ghia, J.E., Khan, W.I., 'Serotonin in the gut: Blessing or a curse?', Biochimie (Jun 2019), 161: 56–64; doi: 10.1016/j.biochi.2018.06.008; Epub 14 Jun 2018; PMID: 29909048

[95] Lee, C.H., Giuliani, F., 'The Role of Inflammation in Depression and Fatigue', Front Immunol (19 Jul 2019), 10: 1696; doi: 10.3389/ fimmu.2019.01696; PMID: 31379879; PMCID: PMC 6658985

[96] Foster, J.A., McVey Neufeld, K.A., 'Gut-brain axis: how the microbiome influences anxiety and depression', Trends Neurosci (May 2013), 36(5): 305–12; doi: 10.1016/j.tins.2013.01.005; Epub 4 Feb 2013; PMID: 23384445

[97] Bermúdez-Humarán, L.G., Salinas, E, Ortiz, G.G. et al., 'From Probiotics to Psychobiotics: Live Beneficial Bacteria Which Act on the Brain–Gut Axis', Nutrients (20 Apr 2019), 11(4): 890; doi: 10.3390/nu11040890; PMID: 31010014; PMCID: PMC 6521058

[98] Bowler, D.E., Buyung-Ali, L.M., Knight, T.M., Pullin, A.S., 'A systematic review of evidence for the added benefits to health of exposure to natural environments', BMC Public Health (2010), 10

[99] Rebar, A.L, Stanton, R., Geard, D. et al., 'A meta-meta-analysis of the effect of physical activity on depression and anxiety in non-clinical adult populations', Health Psychol Rev (2015), 9(3): 366–78

[100] Chen, M.N., Lin, C.C., Liu, C.F., 'Efficacy of phytoestrogens for menopausal symptoms: a meta-analysis and systematic review', Climacteric (Apr 2015), 18(2): 260–9; doi: 10.3109/13697137.2014.966241; Epub 1 Dec 2014; PMID: 25263312; PMCID: PMC4389700

[101] Lai, J., Moxey, A., Nowak, G. et al, 'The efficacy of zinc supplementation in depression: systematic review of randomised controlled trials', J Affect Disord (Jan 2012), 136(1–2): e3–e39; doi: 10.1016/j.jad.2011.06.022; Epub 17 Jul 2011; PMID: 21798601

[102] Derom, M.L., Sayón-Orea, C., Martínez-Ortega, J.M., Martínez-González, M.A., 'Magnesium and depression:

a systematic review', Nutr Neurosci (Sep 2013), 16(5): 191–206; doi: 10.1179/1476830512Y.0000000044; Epub 6 Dec 2012; PMID: 23321048

[103] Patrick, R.P., Ames, B.N., 'Vitamin D hormone regulates serotonin synthesis. Part 1: relevance for autism', FASEB J (Jun 2014), 28(6): 2398–413; doi: 10.1096/fj.13-246546; Epub 20 Feb 2014; PMID: 24558199

[104] Ramaholimihaso T, Bouazzaoui F, Kalajian A. Curcumin, 'Depression: Potential Mechanisms of Action and Current Evidence – A Narrative Review', Front Psychiatry (27 Nov 2020), 11:572533; doi: 10.3389/fpsyt.2020.572533; PMID: 33329109; PMCID: PMC 7728608

[105] Grosso, G., Pajak, A., Marventano, S. et al., 'Role of omega-3 fatty acids in the treatment of depressive disorders: a comprehensive meta-analysis of randomized clinical trials', PLoS One (7 May 2014), 9(5): e96905; doi: 10.1371/journal.pone.0096905; PMID: 24805797; PMCID: PMC4013121

[106] Barton, J., Pretty, J., 'What is the best dose of nature and green exercise for improving mental health? A multi-study analysis', Environ Sci Technol (2010), 44(10): 3947–55

[107] Reddy, N., Desai, M.N., Schoenbrunner, A. et al., 'The complex relationship between estrogen and migraines: a scoping review', Syst Rev (10 Mar 2021), 10(1): 72; doi: 10.1186/s13643-021-01618-4; PMID: 33691790; PMCID: PMC7948327

[108] Wei, P., Liu, M., Chen, Y., Chen, D.C., 'Systematic review of soy isoflavone supplements on osteoporosis in women', Asian Pac J Trop Med (Mar 2012),5(3): 243–8; doi: 10.1016/S1995-7645(12)60033- 9; PMID: 22305793

[109] Kanadys, W., Barańska, A., Błaszczuk, A. et al., 'Effects of Soy Isoflavones on Biochemical Markers of Bone Metabolism in Postmenopausal Women: A Systematic Review and Meta-Analysis of Randomized Controlled Trials', Int J Environ Res Public Health (17 May 2021), 18(10): 5346; doi: 10.3390/ijerph18105346; PMID: 34067865; PMCID: PMC8156509

[110] Akhlaghi, M., Ghasemi Nasab, M., Riasatian, M., Sadeghi, F., 'Soy isoflavones prevent bone resorption and loss, a systematic review and meta-analysis of randomized controlled trials', Crit Rev Food Sci Nutr (2020), 60(14): 2327–41; doi: 10.1080/10408398.2019.1635078; Epub 10 Jul 2019; PMID: 31290343

[111] Prior, J.C., 'Progesterone for the prevention and treatment of osteoporosis in women', Climacteric (Aug 2018), 21(4): 366–74; doi: 10.1080/13697137.2018.1467400; Epub 2 July 2018; PMID: 29962257

[112] Frassetto, L., Banerjee, T., Powe, N., Sebastian, A., 'Acid Balance, Dietary Acid Load, and Bone Effects: A Controversial Subject', Nutrients (21 Apr 2018), 10(4): 517; doi: 10.3390/ nu10040517; PMID: 29690515; PMCID: PMC5946302

[113] Wallace, T.C., Jun, S., Zou, P. et al., 'Dairy intake is not associated with improvements in bone mineral density or risk of fractures across the menopause transition: data from the Study of Women's Health Across the Nation', Menopause (Aug 2020): 27(8): 879–86; doi: 10.1097/GME.0000000000001555

[114] Kucharska, A., Szmurło, A., Sińska, B., 'Significance of diet in treated and untreated acne vulgaris', Postepy Dermatol Alergol (Apr 2016), 33(2): 81–6; doi: 10.5114/ada.2016.59146; Epub 16 May 2016; PMID: 27279815; PMCID: PMC4884775

[115] Kucharska, Szmurło and Sińska in Postepy Dermatol Alergol, 33(2): 81–6

[116] El-Akawi, Z., Abdel-Latif, N., Abdul-Razzak, K., 'Does the plasma level of vitamins A and E affect acne condition?', Clin Exp Dermatol (May 2006), 31(3):430-4; doi: 10.1111/j.1365- 2230.2006.02106.x; PMID: 16681594

[117] Calder, P.C., 'Omega-3 fatty acids and inflammatory processes', Nutrients (Mar 2010), 2(3): 355–74; doi: 10.3390/nu2030355; Epub 18 Mar 2010; PMID: 22254027; PMCID: PMC3257651

[118] Sowers, M.R., Wildman, R.P., Mancuso, P. et al., 'Change in adipocytokines and ghrelin with menopause', Maturitas (20 Feb 2008), 59(2): 149–57; doi: 10.1016/j.maturitas.2007.12.006; Epub 14 Feb 2008; PMID: 18280066; PMCID: PMC2311418

[119] Boonyaratanakornkit, V., Pateetin, P., 'The role of ovarian sex steroids in metabolic homeostasis, obesity, and postmenopausal breast cancer: molecular mechanisms and therapeutic implications', Biomed Res Int. (2015), 2015: 140196; doi: 10.1155/2015/140196; Epub 19 Mar 2015; PMID: 25866757; PMCID: PMC 4383469

[120] Ishihara, T., Yoshida, M., Arita, M., 'Omega-3 fatty acid-derived mediators that control inflammation and tissue homeostasis', Int Immunol (23 Aug 2019), 31(9): 559–67; doi: 10.1093/intimm/dxz001; PMID: 30772915